Anti-Inflammatory Diet for Beginners

Healing with Food: Easy Recipes and Tips for Reducing Inflammation

Shelly B Morrison

Table of Content

Introduction: Embracing the Anti-Inflammatory Lifestyle

"Let food be thy medicine and medicine be thy food." - *Hippocrates*

Welcome, dear reader, to the delicious world of anti-inflammatory eating! Imagine a life where your meals not only tantalize your taste buds but also heal your body from the inside out. Yes, you heard that right. Food can be your medicine, and it's high time we start treating it as such. So, grab your apron, dust off those cooking utensils, and let's embark on this flavorful journey together.

The Sneaky Villain: Inflammation

Picture inflammation as an overzealous firefighter. It rushes to the scene of a problem in your body, eager to help. But instead of dousing a small flame, it ends up flooding your entire house. Sure, a little inflammation is necessary – it's your body's natural response to injury and infection. But chronic inflammation? That's a whole different beast. It's like having that firefighter live in your house, constantly hosing down every nook and cranny, leading to a damp, moldy mess. Chronic inflammation is linked to a smorgasbord of health issues, including arthritis, heart disease, diabetes, and even cancer. Yikes!

The Anti-Inflammatory Diet: Your Culinary Superpower

Enter the anti-inflammatory diet, your culinary superhero cape. This isn't some fad diet promising you'll lose ten pounds in ten days. No, this is about embracing a sustainable, delicious way of eating that will have your body singing with joy. Imagine meals bursting with vibrant colors, rich flavors, and textures so satisfying you'll forget you're even eating "healthy." The anti-inflammatory diet focuses on whole, unprocessed foods like fruits, vegetables, nuts, seeds, lean proteins, and healthy fats. It's about swapping out the bad guys – refined sugars, processed meats, and trans fats – for nutrient-dense, wholesome goodies.

The 30-Day Meal Plan: What's Cooking?

Now, I can hear you asking, "But where do I start?" Fear not, for I have crafted a 30-day meal plan to guide you on this journey. Think of it as your culinary treasure map, leading you to a healthier, more energized you. Each day, you'll discover new recipes that are as delightful to your taste buds as they are to your body. From energizing breakfasts that kickstart your day to comforting dinners that wrap you in a cozy, anti-inflammatory hug, we've got you covered.

Stocking Up: Pantry Staples and Kitchen Tools

Before we dive into the recipes, let's talk about your pantry. Think of it as your superhero utility belt – stocked with everything you need to tackle inflammation head-on. Here's what you'll want to have on hand:

- Extra Virgin Olive Oil: The good fat that's a heart's best friend.

- Turmeric: The golden spice with anti-inflammatory powers.

- Ginger: A zesty root that adds a kick and fights inflammation.

- Leafy Greens: Spinach, kale, and their green friends are packed with antioxidants.

- Berries: Little bursts of flavor that double as anti-inflammatory warriors.

- Nuts and Seeds: Tiny but mighty, these are perfect for snacking and adding crunch to dishes.

- Whole Grains: Quinoa, brown rice, and oats are your new best friends.

- Lean Proteins: Think chicken, turkey, and fish – say goodbye to processed meats.

- Legumes: Beans and lentils for fiber and protein.

- Herbs and Spices: Basil, rosemary, garlic – flavor and health in every pinch.

Next up, let's talk tools. You don't need a kitchen that would make Gordon Ramsay jealous, but a few essentials will make your cooking adventures smoother:

- Sharp Knives: Because no one has time for dull blades.
- Cutting Boards: One for veggies, one for meat – safety first!
- Blender: Perfect for smoothies, soups, and sneaking in veggies.
- Saucepan and Skillet: Your go-to for most recipes.
- Baking Sheets: For roasting veggies and making healthy snacks.
- Measuring Cups and Spoons: Precision is key.
- Mixing Bowls: Because you can never have too many.

Tips for Getting Started

Ready to dive in? Here are a few tips to help you hit the ground running:

1. Plan Ahead: Take a few minutes each week to plan your meals and snacks. Trust me, your future self will thank you.

2. Batch Cook: Make larger portions and freeze leftovers. It's like having your own healthy TV dinners.

3. Stay Hydrated: Water is your best friend. It helps with digestion and keeps everything running smoothly.

4. Listen to Your Body: Pay attention to how different foods make you feel. Everyone's body is unique, so what works for someone else might not work for you.

5. Have Fun: This is an adventure, not a chore. Experiment with new ingredients, try out different recipes, and most importantly, enjoy the process.

So, are you ready to embrace the anti-inflammatory lifestyle? To transform your kitchen into a hub of health and flavor? To turn every meal into a step towards a healthier you? Then let's get cooking! Remember, this is a journey, not a sprint. Take it one meal at a time, and before you know it, you'll be an anti-inflammatory culinary wizard. Now, let's roll up our sleeves and get started – your taste buds and your body are in for a treat!

Chapter 1: Energizing Anti-Inflammatory Breakfasts

"A good breakfast fuels you up and gets you ready for the day." - Unknown

The Morning Magic: Why Breakfast Matters

Good morning, sunshine! The first rays of the day have just peeked through your window, and your stomach gives you that gentle reminder – it's breakfast time. But wait! Before you reach for that sugary cereal or that quick pastry, let's talk about why a good breakfast, especially an anti-inflammatory one, can set the tone for your entire day.

Starting your day with an anti-inflammatory meal is like giving your body a big, warm hug. It's that loving nudge that tells your system, "Hey, we're in this together. Let's start off strong." A nutrient-packed breakfast not only fuels your body but also helps reduce inflammation, stabilize blood sugar levels, and keep those pesky cravings at bay. Imagine feeling energized, focused, and ready to conquer whatever comes your way – that's the power of a good breakfast!

Quick and Easy Breakfast Tips: Because Mornings Are Busy

Now, I know what you're thinking. Mornings can be a whirlwind – getting ready for work, packing lunches, finding those lost keys. Who has time for a fancy breakfast? Fear not! Here are some tips to help you whip up quick and easy anti-inflammatory breakfasts without breaking a sweat:

- Prep the Night Before: Spend a few minutes in the evening preparing your breakfast. Overnight oats, chia pudding, or even a smoothie prepped and ready in the fridge can save you precious time in the morning.

- Batch Cooking: Make larger batches of breakfast items on the weekends. Muffins, breakfast bars, and even cooked quinoa or rice can be stored and quickly reheated for a hassle-free morning meal.

- Keep It Simple: Sometimes, less is more. A piece of fruit with a handful of nuts or a slice of whole-grain toast with avocado can be both quick and nourishing.

- Blender Magic: Smoothies are a busy person's best friend. Throw in some fruits, veggies, a bit of protein, and a liquid base, and you've got a meal in seconds.

- Portable Options: If you're always on the go, look for breakfasts that are easy to take with you. Think smoothie jars, breakfast wraps, or homemade granola bars.

Turmeric Ginger Smoothie Bowl

Servings: 2   Prep Time: 10 minutes

Ingredients:

- 2 frozen bananas
- 1 cup frozen mango chunks
- 1 cup almond milk (or any plant-based milk)
- 1 tsp ground turmeric
- 1/2 tsp fresh grated ginger (or 1/4 tsp ground ginger)
- 1 tbsp chia seeds
- 1/4 cup fresh blueberries
- 1/4 cup granola
- 1 tbsp coconut flakes

Directions:

1. In a blender, combine the frozen bananas, mango chunks, almond milk, turmeric, and ginger.

2. Blend until smooth and creamy, adding more almond milk if needed to reach your desired consistency.

3. Pour the smoothie mixture into two bowls.

4. Top each bowl with chia seeds, fresh blueberries, granola, and coconut flakes.

5. Serve immediately and enjoy!

Tips:

- Use a high-speed blender to achieve a smooth, creamy texture.

- Add a scoop of protein powder for an extra protein boost.

- Experiment with different toppings like nuts, seeds, or fresh fruits.

Nutritional Benefits:

- Turmeric: Contains curcumin, a powerful anti-inflammatory compound.

- Ginger: Known for its anti-inflammatory and antioxidant effects.

- Bananas and Mango: Provide vitamins, minerals, and fiber.

- Chia Seeds: High in omega-3 fatty acids and fiber.

Blueberry Quinoa Breakfast Bake

Servings: 8   Prep Time: 15 minutes

Cook Time: 30 minutes

Ingredients:

- 1 cup quinoa, rinsed
- 2 cups almond milk
- 2 large eggs
- 1/4 cup honey or maple syrup
- 1 tsp vanilla extract
- 1/2 tsp ground cinnamon
- 1/2 tsp baking powder
- 1 cup fresh or frozen blueberries
- 1/4 cup chopped nuts (optional)

Directions:

1. Preheat your oven to 350°F (175°C). Grease a 9x9-inch baking dish.

2. Cook the quinoa according to package instructions.

3. In a large bowl, whisk together the almond milk, eggs, honey, vanilla extract, cinnamon, and baking powder.

4. Stir in the cooked quinoa and blueberries (reserve some blueberries for topping).

5. Pour the mixture into the prepared baking dish and sprinkle with reserved blueberries and nuts.

6. Bake for 30 minutes or until set and golden.

7. Let it cool slightly before slicing into squares.

Tips:

- Store leftovers in the refrigerator and reheat for a quick breakfast.

- Substitute different fruits like raspberries or strawberries for variety.

Nutritional Benefits:

- Quinoa: A complete protein source and rich in fiber.

- Blueberries: High in antioxidants and vitamin C.

- Almond Milk: Low in calories and provides vitamin E.

Avocado Toast with a Twist

Servings: 1   Prep Time: 5 minutes

Ingredients:

- 1 slice whole-grain bread, toasted
- 1/2 ripe avocado
- 1/4 tsp ground turmeric
- 1/4 tsp red pepper flakes
- 1 tsp lemon juice
- Salt and pepper to taste
- Optional toppings: poached egg, cherry tomatoes, microgreens

Directions:

1. Mash the avocado in a small bowl with turmeric, red pepper flakes, lemon juice, salt, and pepper.

2. Spread the mashed avocado mixture over the toasted bread.

3. Top with optional toppings like a poached egg, cherry tomatoes, or microgreens.

4. Serve immediately and enjoy!

Tips:

- Use a ripe avocado for the best texture and flavor.

- Experiment with different spices like cumin or paprika.

- Avocado: Rich in healthy fats and fiber.

- Turmeric: Anti-inflammatory properties.

- Whole-Grain Bread: Provides fiber and nutrients.

Overnight Chia Pudding with Berries

Servings: 2   Prep Time: 10 minutes
+ overnight refrigeration

Ingredients:

- 1/4 cup chia seeds
- 1 cup almond milk (or any plant-based milk)
- 1 tbsp maple syrup or honey
- 1/2 tsp vanilla extract
- 1 cup mixed berries (blueberries, strawberries, raspberries)

1. In a medium bowl, whisk together chia seeds, almond milk, maple syrup, and vanilla extract.

2. Cover and refrigerate overnight or for at least 4 hours.

3. Stir the chia pudding to ensure there are no lumps.

4. Divide the chia pudding into two bowls and top with mixed berries.

5. Serve immediately.

Tips:

- Stir the chia pudding once or twice during the initial hour of refrigeration to prevent clumping.

- Add a dollop of yogurt or a sprinkle of granola for extra texture.

Nutritional Benefits:

- Chia Seeds: High in omega-3 fatty acids, fiber, and protein.

- Berries: Loaded with antioxidants and vitamins.

Sweet Potato Breakfast Hash

Servings: 4   Prep Time: 15 minutes   Cook
Time: 20 minutes

Ingredients:

- 2 medium sweet potatoes, peeled and diced
- 1 red bell pepper, diced
- 1 green bell pepper, diced
- 1 small red onion, diced
- 2 tbsp olive oil
- 1 tsp ground cumin
- 1/2 tsp smoked paprika
- Salt and pepper to taste
- 4 eggs (optional)

Directions:

1. Heat olive oil in a large skillet over medium heat.

2. Add the sweet potatoes, bell peppers, and onion. Season with cumin, smoked paprika, salt, and pepper.

3. Cook, stirring occasionally, until the vegetables are tender and slightly crispy, about 15-20 minutes.

4. If adding eggs, make small wells in the hash and crack an egg into each well. Cover and cook until eggs are set.

5. Serve hot and enjoy!

Tips:

- Use pre-cut vegetables to save time.

- Add a sprinkle of fresh herbs like cilantro or parsley before serving.

Nutritional Benefits:

- Sweet Potatoes: High in beta-carotene, fiber, and vitamins.

- Bell Peppers: Provide vitamin C and antioxidants.

Anti-Inflammatory Green Smoothie

Servings: 2   Prep Time: 5 minutes

Ingredients:

- 1 cup spinach
- 1/2 cup kale
- 1 green apple, cored and chopped
- 1 banana
- 1/2 inch piece of fresh ginger
- 1/2 tsp ground turmeric
- 1 cup coconut water
- 1 tbsp chia seeds

Directions:

1. Combine all ingredients in a blender.

2. Blend until smooth, adding more coconut water if needed to reach desired consistency.

3. Pour into two glasses and serve immediately.

Tips:

- Freeze the banana for a colder, creamier smoothie.

- Adjust the sweetness by adding a bit of honey or another banana.

- Spinach and Kale: Packed with vitamins, minerals, and antioxidants.

- Ginger and Turmeric: Powerful anti-inflammatory agents.

Oatmeal with Cinnamon and Walnuts

Servings: 2   Prep Time: 5 minutes   Cook Time: 10 minutes

Ingredients:

- 1 cup rolled oats
- 2 cups water or almond milk
- 1 tsp ground cinnamon
- 1/4 cup chopped walnuts
- 1 tbsp honey or maple syrup
- Fresh fruit for topping (optional)

Directions:

1. In a medium saucepan, bring the water or almond milk to a boil.

2. Stir in the oats and reduce heat to a simmer.

3. Cook for about 5 minutes, stirring occasionally, until the oats are soft and the liquid is absorbed.

4. Stir in the cinnamon and honey or maple syrup.

5. Divide the oatmeal into two bowls and top with chopped walnuts and fresh fruit.

6. Serve immediately.

Tips:

- Use steel-cut oats for a chewier texture.

- Add a dollop of nut butter for extra protein and creaminess.

Nutritional Benefits:

- Oats: High in fiber and helps lower cholesterol.

- Cinnamon: Has anti-inflammatory and antioxidant properties.

- Walnuts: Rich in omega-3 fatty acids and antioxidants.

Egg Muffins with Spinach and Tomatoes

Servings: 6 muffins   Prep Time: 10 minutes

Cook Time: 20 minutes

Ingredients:

- 6 large eggs
- 1 cup fresh spinach, chopped
- 1/2 cup cherry tomatoes, halved
- 1/4 cup shredded cheese (optional)
- Salt and pepper to taste

Directions:

1. Preheat your oven to 350°F (175°C). Grease a muffin tin with cooking spray.

2. In a large bowl, whisk the eggs and season with salt and pepper.

3. Stir in the chopped spinach, cherry tomatoes, and cheese if using.

4. Pour the egg mixture evenly into the muffin tin cups.

5. Bake for 20 minutes or until the muffins are set and lightly browned.

6. Let cool slightly before removing from the tin. Serve warm.

Tips:

- These can be stored in the refrigerator for up to 5 days and reheated for a quick breakfast.

- Experiment with different veggies and cheese varieties.

Nutritional Benefits:

- Eggs: Excellent source of protein and essential vitamins.

- Spinach and Tomatoes: Provide antioxidants, vitamins, and minerals.

Almond Butter and Banana Toast

Servings: 1   Prep Time: 5 minutes

Ingredients:

- 1 slice whole-grain bread, toasted

- 1 tbsp almond butter

- 1/2 banana, sliced

- 1/2 tsp ground cinnamon

- Drizzle of honey (optional)

Directions:

1. Spread the almond butter over the toasted bread.

2. Arrange the banana slices on top of the almond butter.

3. Sprinkle with ground cinnamon and drizzle with honey if desired.

4. Serve immediately and enjoy!

Tips:

- Use whole-grain or sprouted bread for added nutrients.

- Add a sprinkle of chia seeds or flaxseeds for extra fiber.

Nutritional Benefits:

- Almond Butter: Rich in healthy fats and protein.

- Banana: Provides potassium and natural sweetness.

- Whole-Grain Bread: Offers fiber and complex carbohydrates.

Golden Milk Latte

Servings: 2   Prep Time: 5 minutes   Cook Time: 5 minutes

Ingredients:

- 2 cups almond milk (or any plant-based milk)
- 1 tsp ground turmeric
- 1/2 tsp ground ginger
- 1/2 tsp ground cinnamon
- 1 tbsp honey or maple syrup
- Pinch of black pepper
- 1/2 tsp vanilla extract (optional)

Directions:

1. In a small saucepan, whisk together the almond milk, turmeric, ginger, cinnamon, honey, and black pepper.

2. Heat the mixture over medium heat until it starts to simmer. Do not let it boil.

3. Remove from heat and stir in the vanilla extract if using.

4. Pour into mugs and serve warm.

Tips:

- Use a milk frother for a frothy latte-like texture.

- Adjust the sweetness to your preference with more or less honey.

Nutritional Benefits:

- Turmeric: Known for its potent anti-inflammatory properties.

- Ginger and Cinnamon: Offer additional anti-inflammatory and antioxidant benefits.

- Almond Milk: Low in calories and provides vitamin E.

Chapter 2: Nourishing Anti-Inflammatory Lunches

"Eating a healthy lunch can keep you energized and focused all afternoon." - Unknown

The Power of a Wholesome Lunch

Ah, lunchtime – that midday oasis where you refuel your body and recharge your mind. It's not just about filling your belly; it's about nourishing your body with foods that sustain you through the afternoon slump. When it comes to anti-inflammatory eating, lunch is your opportunity to continue supporting your body's fight against inflammation, all while enjoying delicious meals that keep you satisfied until dinner.

Packing Nutritious Lunches: Your Key to Success

Whether you're heading to the office, school, or simply enjoying a lunch break at home, packing a nutritious lunch sets the tone for the rest of your day. It's the difference between feeling sluggish and distracted or feeling vibrant and focused. With a little planning and creativity, you can pack lunches that are not only anti-inflammatory but also bursting with flavors and textures.

Strategies for Packing Nutritious Lunches:

- Prep Ahead: Spend a bit of time each week prepping ingredients like chopped vegetables, cooked grains, and roasted proteins. This makes assembling lunches during busy mornings a breeze.

- Balance Macronutrients: Aim to include a balance of lean proteins (like chicken, fish, or tofu), healthy fats (avocado, nuts, seeds), and complex carbohydrates (whole grains, legumes) in each meal. This balance helps stabilize blood sugar levels and keeps you full longer.

- Variety is Key: Keep lunches exciting by rotating through different recipes and ingredients. Incorporate a rainbow of vegetables, experiment with different grains and proteins, and don't forget to add fresh herbs and spices for extra flavor and nutrients.

- Packaging Matters: Invest in high-quality containers that keep your food fresh and make it easy to transport. Mason jars are great for salads and layered meals, while bento boxes can keep components separate until you're ready to eat.

Quinoa Salad with Roasted Vegetables

Servings: 4   Prep Time: 15 minutes   Cook Time: 25 minutes

Ingredients:

- 1 cup quinoa, rinsed
- 2 cups water or vegetable broth
- 2 cups mixed vegetables (e.g., bell peppers, zucchini, cherry tomatoes)
- 2 tbsp olive oil
- 1 tsp dried herbs (such as thyme or rosemary)
- Salt and pepper to taste
- Juice of 1 lemon
- 1/4 cup chopped fresh parsley
- Optional: crumbled feta cheese or toasted nuts for garnish

Directions:

1. Preheat your oven to 400°F (200°C). Line a baking sheet with parchment paper.

2. Toss the mixed vegetables with olive oil, dried herbs, salt, and pepper. Spread them evenly on the baking sheet.

3. Roast the vegetables in the preheated oven for about 20-25 minutes, or until they are tender and lightly browned.

4. In the meantime, cook the quinoa according to package instructions.

5. Once cooked, fluff the quinoa with a fork and let it cool slightly.

6. In a large bowl, combine the cooked quinoa and roasted vegetables.

7. Drizzle with lemon juice and toss to combine. Adjust seasoning if needed.

8. Garnish with chopped parsley and optional feta cheese or toasted nuts.

9. Serve warm or chilled.

Tips:

- Use a variety of colorful vegetables for a visually appealing salad.

- Add a protein like grilled chicken or chickpeas for a complete meal.

Nutritional Benefits:

- Quinoa: High in protein, fiber, and essential amino acids.

- Mixed Vegetables: Rich in vitamins, minerals, and antioxidants.

- Olive Oil: Provides healthy fats and anti-inflammatory properties.

Turmeric Chickpea Wraps

Servings: 4   Prep Time: 10 minutes

Cook Time: 10 minutes

Ingredients:

- 1 can (15 oz) chickpeas, drained and rinsed
- 1 tbsp olive oil
- 1 tsp ground turmeric
- 1/2 tsp ground cumin
- Salt and pepper to taste
- 4 whole-grain or gluten-free wraps
- Hummus, for spreading
- Mixed greens or baby spinach
- Sliced cucumber and tomatoes
- Optional: avocado slices, tahini sauce

1. Heat olive oil in a skillet over medium heat.

2. Add the chickpeas, ground turmeric, ground cumin, salt, and pepper. Cook for 5-7 minutes, stirring occasionally, until chickpeas are lightly crispy.

3. Warm the wraps according to package instructions.

4. Spread each wrap with hummus, leaving a border around the edges.

5. Arrange mixed greens or spinach on top of the hummus.

6. Divide the turmeric chickpeas among the wraps, followed by cucumber and tomato slices.

7. Add avocado slices and a drizzle of tahini sauce if desired.

8. Roll up the wraps tightly and slice in half.

9. Serve immediately or wrap tightly in foil for on-the-go lunches.

Tips:

- Customize with your favorite vegetables and spreads.

- Add a squeeze of lemon juice or a sprinkle of paprika for extra flavor.

Nutritional Benefits:

- Chickpeas: Excellent source of plant-based protein and fiber.

- Turmeric: Anti-inflammatory and antioxidant properties.

- Whole-Grain Wraps: Provide fiber and sustained energy.

Grilled Salmon Salad with Avocado

Servings: 2   Prep Time: 10 minutes   Cook Time:
10 minutes

Ingredients:

- 2 salmon fillets
- 1 tbsp olive oil
- Salt and pepper to taste
- Mixed salad greens
- 1 avocado, sliced
- 1/2 cup cherry tomatoes, halved
- 1/4 cup sliced red onion
- Dressing of choice (lemon vinaigrette or balsamic)

Directions:

1. Preheat your grill or grill pan over medium-high heat.

2. Brush salmon fillets with olive oil and season with salt and pepper.

3. Grill the salmon for 4-5 minutes per side, or until cooked through and flaky.

4. Meanwhile, prepare the salad greens and arrange them on plates.

5. Top with sliced avocado, cherry tomatoes, and red onion.

6. Once cooked, place the grilled salmon fillets on top of the salad.

7. Drizzle with your favorite dressing or a squeeze of lemon juice.

8. Serve immediately.

Tips:

- For added flavor, marinate the salmon in lemon juice and herbs before grilling.

- Substitute salmon with grilled chicken or tofu for a different protein option.

Nutritional Benefits:

- Salmon: Rich in omega-3 fatty acids, which have anti-inflammatory effects.

- Avocado: Provides healthy fats and fiber.

- Leafy Greens and Vegetables: Packed with vitamins, minerals, and antioxidants.

Lentil Soup with Spinach

Servings: 6   Prep Time: 10 minutes   Cook Time: 30 minutes

Ingredients:

- 1 cup dried lentils, rinsed
- 1 tbsp olive oil
- 1 onion, chopped
- 2 carrots, diced
- 2 celery stalks, diced
- 3 garlic cloves, minced
- 1 tsp ground cumin
- 1/2 tsp ground turmeric
- 6 cups vegetable broth
- 2 cups fresh spinach, chopped
- Salt and pepper to taste
- Fresh lemon juice for serving
- Optional: chopped fresh parsley for garnish

1. Heat olive oil in a large pot over medium heat.

2. Add the chopped onion, carrots, and celery. Cook for 5-7 minutes, or until vegetables are softened.

3. Stir in the minced garlic, ground cumin, and ground turmeric. Cook for another minute until fragrant.

4. Add the rinsed lentils and vegetable broth to the pot. Bring to a boil.

5. Reduce heat to low, cover, and simmer for 20-25 minutes, or until lentils are tender.

6. Stir in the chopped spinach and cook for 2-3 minutes until wilted.

7. Season with salt and pepper to taste.

8. Serve hot, with a squeeze of fresh lemon juice and garnished with chopped parsley if desired.

Tips:

- Blend half of the soup for a creamier texture, then mix it back with the rest.

- Add a dollop of yogurt or a sprinkle of nutritional yeast for extra creaminess and flavor.

Nutritional Benefits:

- Lentils: High in protein, fiber, and essential nutrients.

- Spinach: Rich in iron, vitamins, and antioxidants.

- Turmeric and Cumin: Provide anti-inflammatory properties.

Mediterranean Chicken Bowl

Servings: 2   Prep Time: 15 minutes   Cook Time: 20 minutes

Ingredients:

- 2 boneless, skinless chicken breasts
- 2 tbsp olive oil, divided
- Salt and pepper to taste
- 1 cup cooked quinoa or brown rice
- 1 cup cherry tomatoes, halved
- 1/2 cucumber, diced
- 1/4 cup Kalamata olives, sliced
- 1/4 cup crumbled feta cheese
- Fresh parsley for garnish
- Dressing of choice (lemon herb or Greek yogurt dressing)

Directions:

1. Preheat your grill or grill pan over medium-high heat.

2. Rub the chicken breasts with 1 tbsp olive oil and season with salt and pepper.

3. Grill the chicken for 6-7 minutes per side, or until cooked through and no longer pink in the center.

4. Let the chicken rest for a few minutes before slicing into strips.

5. In a large bowl, assemble the bowls by dividing cooked quinoa or brown rice between two bowls.

6. Arrange cherry tomatoes, diced cucumber, Kalamata olives, and sliced chicken on top.

7. Sprinkle with crumbled feta cheese and fresh parsley.

8. Drizzle with your favorite dressing or lemon herb sauce.

9. Serve immediately.

Tips:

- Marinate the chicken in lemon juice, olive oil, and Mediterranean herbs for extra flavor.

- Substitute chicken with grilled tofu or chickpeas for a vegetarian option.

Nutritional Benefits:

- Chicken: Lean protein source.

- Quinoa or Brown Rice: Provides fiber and sustained energy.

- Vegetables and Olives: Rich in vitamins, minerals, and antioxidants.

Sweet Potato and Black Bean Tacos

Servings: 4   Prep Time: 15 minutes   Cook Time: 30 minutes

Ingredients:

- 2 large sweet potatoes, peeled and diced
- 1 tbsp olive oil
- 1 tsp ground cumin
- 1/2 tsp smoked paprika
- Salt and pepper to taste
- 1 can (15 oz) black beans, drained and rinsed
- 8 small corn or whole-grain tortillas
- Toppings: avocado slices, salsa, chopped cilantro, lime wedges

1. Preheat your oven to 400°F (200°C). Line a baking sheet with parchment paper.

2. Toss the diced sweet potatoes with olive oil, ground cumin, smoked paprika,

 Salt, and pepper.

3. Spread them in a single layer on the baking sheet and roast for 25-30 minutes, or until tender and lightly browned.

4. In a small saucepan, heat the black beans over medium heat until warmed through.

5. Warm the tortillas in a dry skillet or microwave according to package instructions.

6. To assemble the tacos, fill each tortilla with roasted sweet potatoes and black beans.

7. Top with avocado slices, salsa, chopped cilantro, and a squeeze of lime juice.

8. Serve warm and enjoy!

Tips:

- Add a dollop of Greek yogurt or a sprinkle of cheese for extra creaminess.

- Substitute sweet potatoes with butternut squash or pumpkin for variation.

Nutritional Benefits:

- Sweet Potatoes: Rich in vitamins, minerals, and fiber.

- Black Beans: Excellent source of plant-based protein and fiber.

- Whole-Grain Tortillas: Provide fiber and essential nutrients.

Anti-Inflammatory Buddha Bowl

Servings: 2   Prep Time: 15 minutes   Cook Time: 20 minutes

Ingredients:

- 1 cup quinoa, rinsed
- 2 cups water or vegetable broth
- 1 bunch kale, stems removed and chopped
- 1 sweet potato, peeled and diced
- 1 tbsp olive oil
- Salt and pepper to taste
- 1 avocado, sliced
- 1/4 cup hummus
- 1/4 cup sauerkraut or fermented vegetables
- Optional: sesame seeds or nutritional yeast for garnish

Directions:

1. In a medium pot, combine quinoa and water or vegetable broth. Bring to a boil, then reduce heat to low, cover, and simmer for 15-20 minutes, or until quinoa is cooked and liquid is absorbed.

2. While the quinoa is cooking, preheat your oven to 400°F (200°C). Line a baking sheet with parchment paper.

3. Toss the diced sweet potato with olive oil, salt, and pepper. Spread them in a single layer on the baking sheet.

4. Roast sweet potatoes for 20 minutes, or until tender and lightly browned, flipping halfway through.

5. In a separate skillet, heat a drizzle of olive oil over medium heat. Add chopped kale and sauté for 3-5 minutes, until wilted.

6. To assemble the Buddha bowls, divide cooked quinoa between two bowls.

7. Arrange roasted sweet potatoes, sautéed kale, sliced avocado, hummus, and sauerkraut or fermented vegetables in sections on top of the quinoa.

8. Sprinkle with sesame seeds or nutritional yeast if desired.

9. Serve immediately, drizzled with your favorite dressing or a squeeze of lemon juice.

Tips:

- Customize with your favorite vegetables, beans, or protein sources.

- Batch cook quinoa and roasted sweet potatoes for easy meal prep.

Nutritional Benefits:

- Quinoa: High in protein, fiber, and essential amino acids.

- Kale and Sweet Potatoes: Provide vitamins, minerals, and antioxidants.

- Avocado and Hummus: Rich in healthy fats and fiber.

Spicy Hummus and Veggie Wrap

Servings: 2   Prep Time: 10 minutes

Ingredients:

- 2 large whole-grain or gluten-free wraps

- 1/2 cup spicy hummus

- 1 cup mixed salad greens

- 1/2 cucumber, thinly sliced

- 1/2 bell pepper, thinly sliced

- 1/4 cup shredded carrots

- 1/4 cup alfalfa sprouts or microgreens

Directions:

1. Lay out the wraps on a clean surface.

2. Spread each wrap with 1/4 cup of spicy hummus, leaving a border around the edges.

3. Layer mixed salad greens, sliced cucumber, bell pepper, shredded carrots, and alfalfa sprouts or microgreens evenly over the hummus.

4. Fold in the sides of the wraps and roll tightly.

5. Slice each wrap in half diagonally.

6. Serve immediately or wrap tightly in foil for on-the-go lunches.

Tips:

- Add sliced avocado or a sprinkle of feta cheese for extra flavor and creaminess.

- Use a flavored hummus for variety, such as roasted red pepper or garlic.

Nutritional Benefits:

- Whole-Grain Wraps: Provide fiber and essential nutrients.

- Hummus: Rich in plant-based protein and healthy fats.

- Vegetables: Packed with vitamins, minerals, and antioxidants.

Kale and Apple Salad with Walnuts

Servings: 4   Prep Time: 15 minutes

Ingredients:

- 1 bunch kale, stems removed and chopped
- 1 apple, thinly sliced
- 1/2 cup walnuts, toasted and chopped
- 1/4 cup dried cranberries or raisins
- Juice of 1 lemon
- 2 tbsp olive oil
- 1 tbsp honey or maple syrup (optional)
- Salt and pepper to taste

Directions:

1. In a large bowl, massage the chopped kale with lemon juice and olive oil for 1-2 minutes, until kale begins to soften.

2. Add thinly sliced apple, toasted walnuts, and dried cranberries or raisins to the bowl.

3. Drizzle with honey or maple syrup if using.

4. Toss salad ingredients together until evenly combined.

5. Season with salt and pepper to taste.

6. Serve immediately, or refrigerate for up to 1 hour to allow flavors to meld.

- Massaging kale helps to tenderize it and reduce bitterness.

- Add crumbled goat cheese or feta for a creamy texture and tangy flavor.

Nutritional Benefits:

- Kale: Rich in vitamins A, C, and K, as well as fiber and antioxidants.

- Apples and Walnuts: Provide vitamins, minerals, and healthy fats.

- Dried Cranberries: Add sweetness and additional antioxidants.

Curried Cauliflower Rice

Servings: 4   Prep Time: 10 minutes   Cook Time: 15 minutes

Ingredients:

- 1 head cauliflower, grated or processed into rice-sized pieces
- 2 tbsp coconut oil or olive oil
- 1 onion, finely chopped
- 2 garlic cloves, minced
- 1 tbsp curry powder
- 1/2 tsp ground turmeric
- Salt and pepper to taste
- 1/4 cup chopped fresh cilantro
- Optional: toasted coconut flakes or sliced almonds for garnish

Directions:

1. Grate or process cauliflower into rice-sized pieces using a food processor or box grater.

2. Heat coconut oil or olive oil in a large skillet over medium heat.

3. Add finely chopped onion and minced garlic. Sauté for 3-4 minutes until softened and fragrant.

4. Stir in curry powder and ground turmeric, cooking for an additional minute.

5. Add grated cauliflower to the skillet, stirring to combine with the spices and onion mixture.

6. Cook cauliflower rice for 5-7 minutes, stirring occasionally, until tender but still slightly crisp.

7. Season with salt and pepper to taste.

8. Remove from heat and stir in chopped fresh cilantro.

9. Garnish with toasted coconut flakes or sliced almonds if desired.

10. Serve hot as a side dish or main course.

Tips:

- Use pre-packaged cauliflower rice to save on prep time.

- Add cooked chickpeas or tofu for added protein.

- Cauliflower: Low in calories and carbohydrates, high in fiber and vitamins.

- Curry Powder and Turmeric: Provide anti-inflammatory and antioxidant benefits.

- Coconut Oil: Contains healthy fats and adds a rich flavor.

Chapter 3: Satisfying Anti-Inflammatory Dinners

"Dinner is not just a meal; it's a ritual that brings families together." - Unknown

Embracing the Evening Ritual

As the day winds down, dinner becomes more than just nourishment—it's a time to unwind, connect with loved ones, and savor the flavors of a well-prepared meal. For those embracing the anti-inflammatory lifestyle, dinner presents an opportunity to indulge in dishes that not only satisfy the palate but also support overall health and well-being.

Importance of Ending the Day with a Balanced Meal

A satisfying dinner is crucial for replenishing energy levels, preparing for restful sleep, and ensuring your body receives essential nutrients after a busy day. When crafted with anti-inflammatory ingredients, dinners can help reduce inflammation, support digestive health, and contribute to long-term wellness.

Tips for Meal Prepping Dinners

Meal prepping dinners can streamline your weeknights, making it easier to stick to your anti-inflammatory goals while saving time and effort. Here are some tips to help you get started:

- Plan Ahead: Spend some time each weekend planning your dinners for the upcoming week. This allows you to create balanced meals and ensures you have all necessary ingredients on hand.

- Batch Cooking: Prepare larger batches of grains, proteins (such as grilled chicken or roasted vegetables), and sauces that can be used in multiple meals throughout the week.

- Storage Solutions: Invest in high-quality containers that keep your prepped ingredients fresh. Mason jars are great for salads or layered meals, while glass containers with compartments are ideal for storing different components of your dinner.

- Label and Organize: Label your meal prepped containers with the dish and date to keep track of freshness. Organize your refrigerator so that dinner ingredients are easily accessible when it's time to cook.

Baked Lemon Herb Chicken

Servings: 4   Prep Time: 10 minutes   Cook Time: 30 minutes

Ingredients:

- 4 boneless, skinless chicken breasts
- 2 tbsp olive oil
- Juice of 1 lemon
- Zest of 1 lemon
- 2 garlic cloves, minced
- 1 tsp dried thyme
- 1 tsp dried rosemary
- Salt and pepper to taste
- Fresh herbs (such as parsley or thyme) for garnish

Directions:

1. Preheat your oven to 400°F (200°C). Grease a baking dish lightly with olive oil.

2. In a small bowl, whisk together olive oil, lemon juice, lemon zest, minced garlic, dried thyme, dried rosemary, salt, and pepper.

3. Place the chicken breasts in the prepared baking dish. Pour the lemon herb marinade over the chicken, turning to coat evenly.

4. Bake for 25-30 minutes, or until the chicken is cooked through and reaches an internal temperature of 165°F (75°C).

5. Garnish with fresh herbs before serving.

6. Serve hot with your choice of side dishes like roasted vegetables or quinoa.

Tips:

- Marinate the chicken for a few hours or overnight for enhanced flavor.

- Use a meat thermometer to ensure the chicken is fully cooked without drying out.

Nutritional Benefits:

- Chicken: Lean protein source.

- Lemon and Herbs: Provide antioxidants and add refreshing flavor.

- Olive Oil: Contains healthy fats with anti-inflammatory properties.

Ginger Garlic Shrimp Stir-Fry

Servings: 4   Prep Time: 15 minutes

Cook Time: 10 minutes

Ingredients:

- 1 lb shrimp, peeled and deveined
- 2 tbsp olive oil
- 3 garlic cloves, minced
- 1 tbsp grated fresh ginger
- 1 red bell pepper, thinly sliced
- 1 yellow bell pepper, thinly sliced
- 1 cup snow peas, trimmed
- 2 tbsp low-sodium soy sauce or tamari
- 1 tbsp honey or maple syrup
- Juice of 1 lime
- Salt and pepper to taste
- Fresh cilantro or green onions for garnish

Directions:

1. Heat olive oil in a large skillet or wok over medium-high heat.

2. Add minced garlic and grated ginger, stir-frying for 1 minute until fragrant.

3. Add shrimp to the skillet and cook for 2-3 minutes per side, until pink and cooked through. Remove shrimp from the skillet and set aside.

4. In the same skillet, add sliced bell peppers and snow peas. Stir-fry for 3-4 minutes until vegetables are tender-crisp.

5. Return the shrimp to the skillet. Add soy sauce or tamari, honey or maple syrup, and lime juice. Toss to coat evenly.

6. Season with salt and pepper to taste.

7. Garnish with fresh cilantro or green onions before serving.

8. Serve hot over brown rice or quinoa.

Tips:

- Customize with additional vegetables like broccoli or mushrooms.

- Adjust the sweetness and saltiness of the sauce to suit your taste.

Nutritional Benefits:

- Shrimp: Low in fat and calories, high in protein and essential nutrients.

- Ginger and Garlic: Have anti-inflammatory and immune-boosting properties.

- Bell Peppers and Snow Peas: Provide vitamins, minerals, and antioxidants.

Stuffed Bell Peppers with Quinoa and Veggies

Servings: 4   Prep Time: 20 minutes

Cook Time: 30 minutes

Ingredients:

- 4 bell peppers (any color), tops cut off and seeds removed
- 1 cup quinoa, rinsed
- 2 cups vegetable broth or water
- 1 tbsp olive oil
- 1 onion, chopped
- 2 garlic cloves, minced
- 1 zucchini, diced
- 1 cup cherry tomatoes, halved
- 1 tsp dried oregano
- 1/2 tsp smoked paprika
- Salt and pepper to taste
- 1/4 cup chopped fresh parsley or basil
- Optional: shredded mozzarella or feta cheese

Directions:

1. Preheat your oven to 375°F (190°C). Grease a baking dish with olive oil.

2. In a medium pot, bring vegetable broth or water to a boil. Add quinoa, reduce heat to low, cover, and simmer for 15 minutes, or until quinoa is cooked and liquid is absorbed.

3. Heat olive oil in a large skillet over medium heat. Add chopped onion and minced garlic, sautéing for 3-4 minutes until softened.

4. Add diced zucchini and halved cherry tomatoes to the skillet. Cook for 5-6 minutes until vegetables are tender.

5. Stir in cooked quinoa, dried oregano, smoked paprika, salt, and pepper. Mix well to combine all ingredients.

6. Remove from heat and stir in chopped fresh parsley or basil.

7. Spoon the quinoa and vegetable mixture evenly into the hollowed-out bell peppers.

8. Place stuffed bell peppers in the prepared baking dish. Cover with foil and bake for 20-25 minutes, or until peppers are tender.

9. If using cheese, remove foil during the last 5 minutes of baking to allow cheese to melt and slightly brown.

10. Serve hot, garnished with additional herbs if desired.

Tips:

- Choose firm bell peppers that can stand upright in the baking dish.

- Experiment with different herbs and spices for varied flavors.

Nutritional Benefits:

- Bell Peppers: High in vitamin C and antioxidants.

- Quinoa: Provides complete protein and fiber.

- Zucchini and Cherry Tomatoes: Rich in vitamins, minerals, and water content.

Turmeric-Spiced Lentil Curry

Servings: 6 Prep Time: 15 minutes Cook Time: 30 minutes

Ingredients:

- 1 cup dried lentils, rinsed
- 3 cups vegetable broth
- 1 tbsp olive oil
- 1 onion, finely chopped
- 3 garlic cloves, minced
- 1 tbsp grated fresh ginger
- 1 tbsp curry powder
- 1 tsp ground turmeric
- 1 can (14 oz) diced tomatoes
- 1 can (14 oz) coconut milk
- Salt and pepper to taste
- Fresh cilantro for garnish

Directions:

1. In a large pot, heat olive oil over medium heat. Add chopped onion and sauté for 3-4 minutes until softened.

2. Add minced garlic, grated ginger, curry powder, and ground turmeric to the pot. Cook for 1-2 minutes until fragrant.

3. Stir in rinsed lentils, vegetable broth, diced tomatoes (with their juices), and coconut milk. Bring to a boil.

4. Reduce heat to low, cover, and simmer for 20-25 minutes, or until lentils are tender and cooked through.

5. Season with salt and pepper to taste.

6. Remove from heat and let the curry sit for a few minutes to thicken.

7. Serve hot over cooked brown rice or quinoa.

8. Garnish with fresh cilantro before serving.

Tips:

- Add diced vegetables like carrots, bell peppers, or spinach for extra nutrition.

- Adjust the spice level by adding more or less curry powder and ground turmeric.

- Lentils: Excellent source of plant-based protein, fiber, and essential nutrients.

- Turmeric and Ginger: Have potent anti-inflammatory and antioxidant properties.

- Coconut Milk: Adds creaminess and healthy fats.

Balsamic Glazed Salmon

Servings: 4   Prep Time: 10 minutes

Cook Time: 15 minutes

Ingredients:

- 4 salmon fillets
- 2 tbsp olive oil
- Salt and pepper to taste
- 1/4 cup balsamic vinegar
- 2 tbsp honey or maple syrup
- 2 garlic cloves, minced
- Fresh parsley for garnish

Directions:

1. Preheat your oven to 400°F (200°C). Line a baking sheet with parchment paper.

2. Place salmon fillets on the prepared baking sheet. Drizzle with olive oil and season with salt and pepper.

3. In a small saucepan, combine balsamic vinegar, honey or maple syrup, and minced garlic. Bring to a simmer over medium heat.

4. Cook the glaze for 3-4 minutes, stirring occasionally, until it thickens slightly.

5. Brush half of the balsamic glaze over the salmon fillets.

6. Bake salmon for 12-15 minutes, or until fish flakes easily with a fork.

7. Remove from the oven and brush with remaining balsamic glaze.

8. Garnish with fresh parsley before serving.

- Broil the salmon for the last 1-2 minutes to caramelize the glaze.

- Serve with roasted vegetables or a side salad for a complete meal.

Nutritional Benefits:

- Salmon: Rich in omega-3 fatty acids, which have anti-inflammatory effects.

- Balsamic Vinegar: Provides antioxidants and adds a sweet-tangy flavor.

- Honey or Maple Syrup: Natural sweeteners with potential health benefits.

Zucchini Noodles with Pesto and Cherry Tomatoes

Servings: 4   Prep Time: 15 minutes

Cook Time: 10 minutes

- 4 medium zucchini, spiralized into noodles

- 1 cup cherry tomatoes, halved

- 1/2 cup basil pesto (store-bought or homemade)

- 2 tbsp olive oil

- 2 garlic cloves, minced

- Salt and pepper to taste

- Grated Parmesan cheese (optional) for garnish

Directions:

1. Heat olive oil in a large skillet over medium heat. Add minced garlic and cook for 1 minute until fragrant.

2. Add cherry tomatoes to the skillet and cook for 2-3 minutes until they start to soften.

3. Add zucchini noodles to the skillet and toss gently with tongs. Cook for 3-4 minutes until zucchini noodles are tender but still al dente.

4. Remove skillet from heat and stir in basil pesto until zucchini noodles are evenly coated.

5. Season with salt and pepper to taste.

6. Divide zucchini noodles and cherry tomatoes among serving plates.

7. Garnish with grated Parmesan cheese if desired.

8. Serve immediately, optionally with grilled chicken or shrimp on top.

Tips:

- Pat zucchini noodles dry with paper towels to remove excess moisture before cooking.

- Add pine nuts or walnuts to the pesto for extra texture and flavor.

Nutritional Benefits:

- Zucchini: Low in calories and carbohydrates, high in fiber and vitamins.

- Cherry Tomatoes: Provide vitamins, minerals, and antioxidants.

- Basil Pesto: Contains healthy fats from olive oil and pine nuts, plus anti-inflammatory properties from basil.

Roasted Brussels Sprouts and Sweet Potatoes

Servings: 4   Prep Time: 10 minutes   Cook Time: 30 minutes

Ingredients:

- 1 lb Brussels sprouts, trimmed and halved
- 2 medium sweet potatoes, peeled and diced
- 2 tbsp olive oil
- 1 tsp garlic powder
- 1 tsp smoked paprika
- Salt and pepper to taste
- Optional: balsamic glaze or honey for drizzling
- Fresh parsley or thyme for garnish

Directions:

1. Preheat your oven to 400°F (200°C). Line a baking sheet with parchment paper.

2. In a large bowl, toss Brussels sprouts and diced sweet potatoes with olive oil, garlic powder, smoked paprika, salt, and pepper until evenly coated.

3. Spread vegetables in a single layer on the prepared baking sheet.

4. Roast for 25-30 minutes, stirring halfway through, until Brussels sprouts are crispy and sweet potatoes are tender.

5. Remove from the oven and drizzle with balsamic glaze or honey if desired.

6. Garnish with fresh parsley or thyme before serving.

Tips:

- Cut Brussels sprouts into halves or quarters for quicker cooking.

- Add chopped pecans or almonds during the last 10 minutes of roasting for extra crunch.

Nutritional Benefits:

- Brussels Sprouts: Rich in fiber, vitamins C and K, and antioxidants.

- Sweet Potatoes: Provide vitamins, minerals, and complex carbohydrates.

- Olive Oil and Spices: Offer heart-healthy fats and anti-inflammatory properties.

Chicken and Vegetable Skewers

Servings: 4   Prep Time: 20 minutes (plus 30 minutes marinating time)

Cook Time: 10 minutes

Ingredients:

- 1 lb boneless, skinless chicken breasts, cut into cubes
- 1 zucchini, sliced into rounds
- 1 red bell pepper, cut into chunks
- 1 yellow bell pepper, cut into chunks
- 1 red onion, cut into chunks
- 1/4 cup olive oil
- Juice of 1 lemon
- 2 garlic cloves, minced
- 1 tsp dried oregano
- Salt and pepper to taste
- Wooden or metal skewers

Directions:

1. If using wooden skewers, soak them in water for at least 30 minutes before grilling to prevent burning.

2. In a large bowl, whisk together olive oil, lemon juice, minced garlic, dried oregano, salt, and pepper.

3. Add chicken cubes to the marinade, tossing to coat evenly. Cover and refrigerate for at least 30 minutes, or up to 4 hours.

4. Preheat your grill or grill pan over medium-high heat.

5. Thread marinated chicken, zucchini rounds, bell pepper chunks, and red onion chunks onto skewers, alternating between ingredients.

6. Grill skewers for 4-5 minutes per side, or until chicken is cooked through and vegetables are tender-crisp, with slight char marks.

7. Remove from the grill and let skewers rest for a few minutes before serving.

8. Serve hot with a side of quinoa or couscous.

Tips:

- Use metal skewers for easy cleanup and durability.

- Brush leftover marinade onto skewers while grilling for added flavor.

Nutritional Benefits:

- Chicken: Lean protein source.

- Vegetables: Provide vitamins, minerals, and antioxidants.

- Olive Oil and Lemon: Offer heart-healthy fats and vitamin C.

Anti-Inflammatory Beef Stew

Servings: 6   Prep Time: 20 minutes

Cook Time: 2 hours

Ingredients:

- 1 lb beef stew meat, cubed
- 2 tbsp olive oil
- 1 onion, chopped
- 2 garlic cloves, minced
- 2 carrots, sliced
- 2 celery stalks, sliced
- 1 sweet potato, peeled and diced
- 1 cup diced tomatoes (canned or fresh)
- 4 cups low-sodium beef broth
- 1 tbsp tomato paste
- 1 tsp dried thyme
- 1 tsp dried rosemary

- Salt and pepper to taste

- Fresh parsley for garnish

Directions:

1. In a large pot or Dutch oven, heat olive oil over medium-high heat.

2. Add cubed beef stew meat to the pot and cook for 5-6 minutes until browned on all sides. Remove beef from the pot and set aside.

3. In the same pot, add chopped onion and minced garlic. Sauté for 3-4 minutes until softened.

4. Add sliced carrots, sliced celery, and diced sweet potato to the pot. Cook for 5 minutes, stirring occasionally.

5. Stir in diced tomatoes, beef broth, tomato paste, dried thyme, dried rosemary, salt, and pepper.

6. Return browned beef stew meat to the pot. Bring to a boil, then reduce heat to low.

7. Cover and simmer for 1.5 to 2 hours, stirring occasionally, until beef and vegetables are tender.

8. Season with additional salt and pepper if needed.

9. Remove from heat and let the stew sit for a few minutes to allow flavors to meld.

10. Serve hot, garnished with fresh parsley.

Tips:

- For a thicker stew, mix 1 tbsp cornstarch with 2 tbsp cold water and stir into the stew during the last 10 minutes of cooking.

- Pair with crusty whole-grain bread or brown rice for a complete meal.

Nutritional Benefits:

- Beef: Provides high-quality protein, iron, and essential nutrients.

- Vegetables: Rich in vitamins, minerals, and fiber.

- Broth and Herbs: Enhance flavor and offer additional nutrients.

Spaghetti Squash with Marinara Sauce

Servings: 4   Prep Time: 10 minutes   Cook Time: 45 minutes

Ingredients:

- 1 large spaghetti squash

- 2 tbsp olive oil

- Salt and pepper to taste

- 2 cups marinara sauce (store-bought or homemade)

- Fresh basil leaves for garnish

- Grated Parmesan cheese (optional)

Directions:

1. Preheat your oven to 400°F (200°C). Line a baking sheet with parchment paper.

2. Carefully cut the spaghetti squash in half lengthwise. Scoop out the seeds and discard.

3. Drizzle olive oil over the cut sides of the spaghetti squash halves. Season with salt and pepper.

4. Place the spaghetti squash halves cut-side down on the prepared baking sheet.

5. Bake for 35-45 minutes, or until the squash is tender and easily pierced with a fork.

6. Remove from the oven and let cool for 10 minutes.

7. Use a fork to scrape the flesh of the spaghetti squash into strands.

8. Heat marinara sauce in a saucepan over medium heat until warmed through.

9. Divide spaghetti squash strands among serving plates. Top with marinara sauce.

10. Garnish with fresh basil leaves and grated Parmesan cheese if desired.

11. Serve hot as a nutritious and satisfying pasta alternative.

Tips:

- For extra flavor, roast the spaghetti squash with minced garlic or dried herbs.

- Add cooked lean ground turkey or chicken to the marinara sauce for added protein.

Nutritional Benefits:

- Spaghetti Squash: Low in calories and carbohydrates, high in fiber and vitamins.

- Marinara Sauce: Provides lycopene and other antioxidants from tomatoes.

- Olive Oil and Parmesan Cheese: Offer healthy fats and additional flavor.

Chapter 4: Healing Anti-Inflammatory Snacks

"Snacking can be a healthy part of your diet if done right." - Unknown

Snacking plays a crucial role in maintaining energy levels and preventing overeating during main meals. When following an anti-inflammatory diet, snacks can also serve as an opportunity to incorporate more nutrients and support overall health. This chapter explores delicious and easy-to-prepare snack ideas that are not only satisfying but also contribute to reducing inflammation.

Benefits of Snacking on Anti-Inflammatory Foods

Snacks provide an opportunity to:

Maintain steady blood sugar levels throughout the day.

Boost energy and combat fatigue.

Provide essential nutrients and antioxidants.

Aid in weight management by preventing excessive hunger.

Turmeric Roasted Chickpeas

Servings: 4   Prep Time: 5 minutes   Cook Time: 30 minutes

Ingredients:

- 2 cans (15 oz each) chickpeas, drained, rinsed, and patted dry
- 2 tbsp olive oil
- 1 tsp ground turmeric
- 1/2 tsp ground cumin
- 1/2 tsp smoked paprika
- Salt to taste

Directions:

1. Preheat your oven to 400°F (200°C). Line a baking sheet with parchment paper.

2. In a bowl, toss chickpeas with olive oil, turmeric, cumin, smoked paprika, and salt until evenly coated.

3. Spread chickpeas in a single layer on the prepared baking sheet.

4. Roast for 25-30 minutes, shaking the pan halfway through, until chickpeas are crispy and golden brown.

5. Remove from the oven and let cool slightly before serving.

Tips:

- Pat chickpeas dry with a paper towel to ensure crispiness.

- Experiment with different spice blends like curry powder or garlic powder.

Nutritional Benefits:

- Chickpeas: Excellent source of plant-based protein, fiber, and minerals.

- Turmeric: Contains curcumin, known for its anti-inflammatory properties.

Apple Slices with Almond Butter

Servings: 2   Prep Time: 5 minutes

Ingredients:

- 1 large apple, cored and sliced
- 4 tbsp almond butter

Directions:

1. Arrange apple slices on a plate.

2. Serve with almond butter for dipping or spreading.

Tips:

- Sprinkle apple slices with cinnamon for added flavor.

- Choose organic apples for fewer pesticides.

Nutritional Benefits:

- Apples: High in fiber, vitamins, and antioxidants.

- Almond Butter: Provides protein, healthy fats, and vitamin E.

Cucumber Hummus Bites

Servings: 4   Prep Time: 10 minutes

Ingredients:

- 1 large cucumber, sliced into rounds

- 1/2 cup hummus (store-bought or homemade)

- Fresh parsley or dill for garnish

Directions:

1. Arrange cucumber rounds on a serving platter.

2. Top each cucumber round with a spoonful of hummus.

3. Garnish with fresh parsley or dill.

Tips:

- Use mini cucumbers for bite-sized snacks.

- Add a sprinkle of paprika or black pepper for extra flavor.

Nutritional Benefits:

- Cucumber: Hydrating and low in calories, with vitamins and minerals.

- Hummus: Provides protein, fiber, and essential nutrients.

Mixed Berry Yogurt Parfait

Servings: 2   Prep Time: 5 minutes

Ingredients:

- 1 cup Greek yogurt (unsweetened)
- 1 cup mixed berries (such as blueberries, strawberries, raspberries)
- 2 tbsp honey or maple syrup (optional)
- 1/4 cup granola (optional)

Directions:

1. In serving glasses or bowls, layer Greek yogurt and mixed berries.

2. Drizzle with honey or maple syrup if desired.

3. Top with granola for added crunch.

Tips:

- Choose plain Greek yogurt to avoid added sugars.

- Substitute with dairy-free yogurt for a vegan option.

Nutritional Benefits:

- Greek Yogurt: Rich in probiotics, protein, and calcium.

- Berries: Packed with antioxidants and fiber.

- Honey or Maple Syrup: Natural sweeteners with potential health benefits.

Spiced Pumpkin Seeds

Servings: 4   Prep Time: 5 minutes

Cook Time: 15 minutes

Ingredients:

- 2 cups raw pumpkin seeds (pepitas)
- 1 tbsp olive oil
- 1 tsp ground cumin
- 1/2 tsp smoked paprika
- 1/2 tsp sea salt

Directions:

1. Preheat your oven to 325°F (160°C). Line a baking sheet with parchment paper.

2. In a bowl, toss pumpkin seeds with olive oil, cumin, smoked paprika, and sea salt until evenly coated.

3. Spread pumpkin seeds in a single layer on the prepared baking sheet.

4. Roast for 12-15 minutes, stirring occasionally, until pumpkin seeds are golden and crispy.

5. Remove from the oven and let cool before serving.

Tips:

- Add a pinch of cayenne pepper for a spicy kick.

- Store in an airtight container for up to one week.

Nutritional Benefits:

- Pumpkin Seeds: High in protein, fiber, and healthy fats.

- Cumin and Paprika: Provide antioxidants and anti-inflammatory properties.

- Olive Oil: Enhances flavor and offers heart-healthy fats.

Avocado Deviled Eggs

Servings: 4   Prep Time: 15 minutes   Cook Time: 12 minutes (plus cooling time)

Ingredients:

- 4 large eggs
- 1 ripe avocado
- 1 tbsp Greek yogurt (optional)
- 1 tsp Dijon mustard
- 1 tsp lemon juice
- Salt and pepper to taste
- Paprika for garnish

Directions:

1. Place eggs in a saucepan and cover with cold water. Bring to a boil over medium-high heat.

2. Once boiling, remove from heat, cover, and let eggs sit for 10-12 minutes.

3. Transfer eggs to a bowl of ice water and let cool for 5 minutes. Peel eggs and slice in half lengthwise.

4. Remove yolks and place in a bowl. Mash yolks with avocado, Greek yogurt (if using), Dijon mustard, lemon juice, salt, and pepper until smooth.

5. Spoon or pipe avocado mixture into egg white halves.

6. Sprinkle with paprika for garnish.

Tips:

- Use a ziplock bag with the corner cut off to pipe the avocado mixture into egg whites for a cleaner presentation.

- Serve immediately or refrigerate until ready to serve.

Nutritional Benefits:

- Eggs: Excellent source of protein and essential nutrients.

- Avocado: Provides healthy fats, fiber, and vitamins.

- Greek Yogurt: Adds creaminess and additional protein.

Carrot and Celery Sticks with Tahini Dip

Servings: 4   Prep Time: 10 minutes

Ingredients:

- 2 large carrots, cut into sticks
- 2 celery stalks, cut into sticks
- 1/4 cup tahini
- 2 tbsp lemon juice
- 1 garlic clove, minced
- 1/4 tsp ground cumin
- Salt and pepper to taste
- Water (as needed for thinning)

Directions:

1. Arrange carrot and celery sticks on a serving platter.

2. In a bowl, whisk together tahini, lemon juice, minced garlic, ground cumin, salt, and pepper.

3. Add water gradually, stirring until desired consistency is reached.

4. Serve carrot and celery sticks with tahini dip.

Tips:

- Add a drizzle of olive oil and sprinkle of paprika for extra flavor.

- Refrigerate leftover dip in an airtight container for up to one week.

Nutritional Benefits:

- Carrots and Celery: Low-calorie vegetables high in fiber, vitamins, and antioxidants.

- Tahini: Rich in healthy fats, protein, and minerals.

- Lemon Juice: Provides vitamin C and enhances flavor.

Anti-Inflammatory Trail Mix

Servings: 4   Prep Time: 5 minutes

Ingredients:

- 1 cup mixed nuts (such as almonds, walnuts, cashews)

- 1/2 cup dried cranberries

- 1/4 cup pumpkin seeds

- 1/4 cup dark chocolate chips (optional)

Directions:

1. In a bowl, combine mixed nuts, dried cranberries, pumpkin seeds, and dark chocolate chips if using.

2. Mix well and portion into individual servings or store in an airtight container.

Tips:

- Choose unsweetened and unsalted nuts and seeds for a healthier option.

- Customize with your favorite nuts, seeds, and dried fruits.

Nutritional Benefits:

- Nuts and Seeds: Provide protein, healthy fats, and essential nutrients.

- Dried Cranberries: Add natural sweetness and antioxidants.

- Dark Chocolate: Contains flavonoids with potential health benefits.

Dark Chocolate and Nut Clusters

Servings: 8 clusters   Prep Time: 10 minutes   Cook Time: 5 minutes (plus chilling time)

Ingredients:

- 1/2 cup dark chocolate chips or chunks

- 1 cup mixed nuts (such as almonds, cashews, pistachios)

- Sea salt flakes for sprinkling (optional)

Directions:

1. Line a baking sheet with parchment paper.

2. In a microwave-safe bowl, melt dark chocolate chips in 30-second intervals, stirring in between, until smooth.

3. Stir mixed nuts into melted chocolate until well coated.

4. Drop spoonfuls of chocolate-coated nuts onto the prepared baking sheet, forming clusters.

5. Sprinkle with sea salt flakes if desired.

6. Refrigerate for 30 minutes or until chocolate is set.

Tips:

- Use a double boiler for melting chocolate if you prefer.

- Store clusters in the refrigerator in an airtight container.

Nutritional Benefits:

- Dark Chocolate: Contains antioxidants and may have heart health benefits.

- Mixed Nuts: Provide protein, healthy fats, and essential nutrients.

- Sea Salt: Enhances flavor and provides trace minerals.

Golden Milk Energy Bites

Servings: 12 bites   Prep Time: 15 minutes

Chill Time: 30 minutes

Ingredients:

- 1 cup rolled oats
- 1/2 cup almond butter
- 1/4 cup honey or maple syrup
- 2 tbsp ground flaxseed
- 1 tsp ground turmeric
- 1/2 tsp ground cinnamon
- Pinch of black pepper
- Pinch of sea salt
- 1/4 cup chopped almonds or cashews (optional)

Directions:

1. In a bowl, combine rolled oats, almond butter, honey or maple syrup, ground flaxseed, turmeric, cinnamon, black pepper, sea salt, and chopped nuts if using.

2. Mix until well combined and sticky.

3. Roll mixture into tablespoon-sized balls and place on a baking sheet lined with parchment paper.

4. Chill in the refrigerator for at least 30 minutes before serving.

Tips:

- Add shredded coconut or cocoa powder for extra flavor variations.

- Store energy bites in the refrigerator in an airtight container for up to one week.

Nutritional Benefits:

- Oats and Nuts: Provide fiber, protein, and sustained energy.

- Turmeric: Contains curcumin with anti-inflammatory properties.

- Honey or Maple Syrup: Natural sweeteners with potential health benefits.

Chapter 5: Refreshing Anti-Inflammatory Beverages

"Hydration is key to maintaining overall health." - Unknown

Hydration is essential for supporting bodily functions and maintaining overall health. In an anti-inflammatory diet, beverages play a crucial role not only in hydrating the body but also in providing essential nutrients and antioxidants that help reduce inflammation. This chapter explores a variety of refreshing beverages that are not only delicious but also promote a healthy inflammatory response.

Role of Beverages in an Anti-Inflammatory Diet

Hydrate the body and support optimal cellular function.

Provide antioxidants that combat oxidative stress and inflammation.

Offer vitamins and minerals crucial for overall health and well-being..

-Certainly! Here are detailed recipes for each of the anti-inflammatory beverages:

Ginger Turmeric Tea

Servings: 2   Prep Time: 5 minutes

Cook Time: 10 minutes

Ingredients:

- 2 cups water
- 1-inch piece fresh ginger, thinly sliced
- 1-inch piece fresh turmeric, thinly sliced (or 1 tsp ground turmeric)
- 1-2 tbsp honey or maple syrup (optional)
- Juice of 1/2 lemon (optional)

Directions:

1. In a small saucepan, bring water to a boil.

2. Add ginger and turmeric slices to the boiling water.

3. Reduce heat and simmer for 5-10 minutes.

4. Remove from heat and let steep for an additional 5 minutes.

5. Strain tea into cups. Stir in honey or maple syrup and lemon juice if desired.

6. Serve hot.

Tips:

- Adjust sweetness and strength of flavor by varying the amount of honey or ginger.

- Store leftover tea in the refrigerator and reheat before serving.

Nutritional Benefits:

- Ginger and Turmeric: Both have potent anti-inflammatory and antioxidant properties.

- Honey or Maple Syrup: Natural sweeteners with potential health benefits.

- Lemon: Provides vitamin C and adds a refreshing citrus flavor.

Cucumber Mint Water

Servings: 4   Prep Time: 5 minutes

Ingredients:

- 1 large cucumber, thinly sliced
- 1/4 cup fresh mint leaves
- 6 cups water
- Ice cubes

Directions:

1. In a pitcher, combine cucumber slices and fresh mint leaves.

2. Add water and stir to combine.

3. Refrigerate for at least 1 hour to allow flavors to infuse.

4. Serve over ice.

Tips:

- Use a vegetable peeler to create thin cucumber slices.

- Garnish with additional mint leaves for a more pronounced flavor.

Nutritional Benefits:

- Cucumber: Hydrating and low in calories, with vitamins and minerals.

- Mint: Refreshing herb that aids digestion and adds a crisp flavor.

- Water: Essential for hydration and optimal bodily functions.

Anti-Inflammatory Smoothie

Servings: 2   Prep Time: 5 minutes

Ingredients:

- 1 cup spinach leaves
- 1 cup kale leaves, stems removed
- 1/2 cup frozen pineapple chunks
- 1/2 cup frozen berries (such as blueberries or strawberries)
- 1-inch piece fresh ginger, peeled
- 1-inch piece fresh turmeric, peeled (or 1/2 tsp ground turmeric)
- 1 cup coconut water or almond milk

Directions:

1. In a blender, combine spinach, kale, pineapple, berries, ginger, turmeric, and coconut water or almond milk.

2. Blend until smooth and creamy.

3. Pour into glasses and serve immediately.

Tips:

- Add a banana for extra creaminess and sweetness.

- Adjust consistency with more coconut water or almond milk as needed.

Nutritional Benefits:

- Spinach and Kale: Packed with vitamins, minerals, and antioxidants.

- Pineapple and Berries: Provide natural sweetness and vitamin C.

- Ginger and Turmeric: Anti-inflammatory and immune-boosting properties.

Green Juice with Spinach and Kale

Servings: 2   Prep Time: 10 minutes

Ingredients:

- 2 cups spinach leaves

- 1 cup kale leaves, stems removed

- 1 cucumber, peeled and chopped

- 1 green apple, cored and chopped

- Juice of 1 lemon

- 1-inch piece fresh ginger, peeled

- 1 cup water or coconut water

- Ice cubes (optional)

Directions:

1. In a juicer or blender, process spinach, kale, cucumber, apple, lemon juice, ginger, and water or coconut water until smooth.

2. Strain juice through a fine mesh sieve if desired.

3. Serve over ice cubes if preferred.

Tips:

- Adjust sweetness by adding more apple or a splash of honey.

- Drink immediately for maximum freshness and nutrients.

Nutritional Benefits:

- Spinach and Kale: Rich in vitamins A, C, and K, as well as antioxidants.

- Cucumber: Hydrating and aids in detoxification.

- Apple and Lemon: Provide natural sweetness and vitamin C.

Berry Infused Water

Servings: 4   Prep Time: 5 minutes

Ingredients:

- 1 cup mixed berries (such as strawberries, raspberries, blueberries)
- 8 cups water
- Ice cubes

Directions:

1. In a pitcher, muddle mixed berries slightly to release juices.

2. Add water and stir gently to combine.

3. Refrigerate for at least 1 hour to allow flavors to infuse.

4. Serve over ice cubes.

Tips:

- Use fresh or frozen berries depending on availability.

- Add a sprig of mint or basil for added flavor.

Nutritional Benefits:

- Berries: High in antioxidants and vitamins, supporting immune health.

- Water: Essential for hydration and flushing out toxins.

Golden Milk

Servings: 2   Prep Time: 5 minutes   Cook Time: 10 minutes

Ingredients:

- 2 cups milk (dairy or plant-based)
- 1 tsp ground turmeric
- 1/2 tsp ground cinnamon
- 1/4 tsp ground ginger
- Pinch of black pepper
- 1 tbsp honey or maple syrup (optional)

Directions:

1. In a small saucepan, whisk together milk, turmeric, cinnamon, ginger, and black pepper.

2. Bring mixture to a simmer over medium heat, stirring occasionally.

3. Remove from heat and let cool slightly.

4. Stir in honey or maple syrup if desired.

5. Pour into mugs and serve warm.

Tips:

- Use freshly grated turmeric and ginger for a more intense flavor.

- Adjust sweetness and spices to taste preferences.

Nutritional Benefits:

- Turmeric: Contains curcumin with potent anti-inflammatory properties.

- Cinnamon and Ginger: Provide additional antioxidants and flavor.

- Milk: Offers calcium, vitamin D, and protein.

Lemon Ginger Detox Drink

Servings: 2   Prep Time: 5 minutes

Ingredients:

- 2 cups water
- Juice of 1 lemon
- 1-inch piece fresh ginger, grated
- 1 tbsp honey or maple syrup (optional)
- Ice cubes

Directions:

1. In a pitcher, combine water, lemon juice, grated ginger, and honey or maple syrup.

2. Stir well until honey or maple syrup is dissolved.

3. Refrigerate for at least 30 minutes to allow flavors to meld.

4. Serve over ice cubes.

Tips:

- Add a dash of cayenne pepper for an extra detoxifying boost.

- Drink first thing in the morning for a refreshing start to the day.

- Lemon: Alkalizing and rich in vitamin C.

- Ginger: Supports digestion and has anti-inflammatory properties.

- Honey or Maple Syrup: Provides natural sweetness and potential health benefits.

Pineapple Turmeric Smoothie

Servings:2   Prep Time: 5 minutes

Ingredients:

- 1 cup frozen pineapple chunks
- 1 banana
- 1 cup coconut water or almond milk
- 1 tsp ground turmeric
- 1/2 tsp ground ginger
- 1 tbsp chia seeds (optional)
- Ice cubes

Directions:

1. In a blender, combine frozen pineapple, banana, coconut water or almond milk, turmeric, ginger, and chia seeds if using.

2. Blend until smooth and creamy.

3. Add ice cubes and blend again until desired consistency is reached.

4. Pour into glasses and serve immediately.

Tips:

- Use fresh pineapple and freeze it ahead of time for a colder smoothie.

- Substitute spinach or kale for added greens.

Nutritional Benefits:

- Pineapple: Contains bromelain, an enzyme with anti-inflammatory properties.

- Turmeric and Ginger: Anti-inflammatory and immune-boosting properties.

- Chia Seeds: Provide omega-3 fatty acids and fiber.

Herbal Anti-Inflammatory Iced Tea

Servings: 4   Prep Time: 5 minutes

Cook Time: 10 minutes (plus cooling time)

Ingredients:

- 4 cups water
- 2 tbsp loose herbal tea (such as chamomile, rooibos, or hibiscus)
- 1-inch piece fresh ginger, sliced
- Juice of 1/2 lemon
- Honey or maple syrup to taste (optional)
- Ice cubes

Directions:

1. In a saucepan, bring water to a boil.

2. Remove from heat and add herbal tea and sliced ginger.

3. Let steep for 5-10 minutes, depending on desired strength.

4. Strain tea into a pitcher and let cool to room temperature.

5. Stir in lemon juice and sweeten with honey or maple syrup if desired.

6. Refrigerate until chilled.

7. Serve over ice cubes.

- Adjust the amount of honey or maple syrup based on your sweetness preference.

- Experiment with different herbal tea blends for variety.

Nutritional Benefits:

- Herbal Tea: Contains antioxidants and can have anti-inflammatory effects.

- Ginger: Adds flavor and supports digestive health.

- Lemon: Provides vitamin C and enhances the tea's refreshing taste.

Coconut Water and Aloe Vera Drink

Servings: 2   Prep Time: 5 minutes

Ingredients:

- 1 cup coconut water
- 1/2 cup aloe vera juice (preferably unsweetened)
- Juice of 1 lime
- 1 tbsp honey or agave syrup (optional)
- Ice cubes

Directions:

1. In a blender, combine coconut water, aloe vera juice, lime juice, and honey or agave syrup.

2. Blend until smooth.

3. Serve over ice cubes.

Tips:

- Choose pure aloe vera juice without added sugars for the most health benefits.

- Adjust sweetness and tartness by varying the amount of lime juice and sweetener.

Nutritional Benefits:

- Coconut Water: Hydrating and rich in electrolytes.

- Aloe Vera: Supports digestion and may have anti-inflammatory properties.

- Lime: Provides vitamin C and adds a refreshing citrus flavor.

Chapter 6: Comforting Anti-Inflammatory Soups and Stews

"A bowl of soup can warm the soul and nourish the body." -
Unknown

Soups and stews have long been cherished for their ability to comfort and heal. In an anti-inflammatory diet, they offer a perfect way to pack a variety of nutrients and flavors into one satisfying meal. This chapter explores the benefits of soups and stews, along with tips for creating hearty and healthy recipes.

Benefits of Soups and Stews in an Anti-Inflammatory Diet

Soups and stews: Provide hydration and warmth, supporting overall well-being.

Allow for easy incorporation of anti-inflammatory ingredients like turmeric, ginger, and leafy greens.

Are versatile and can be tailored to include a wide range of vegetables, legumes, and lean proteins.

Tips for Making Hearty and Healthy Soups

Use a flavorful base: Start with a homemade vegetable or bone broth to enhance the depth of flavor. Incorporate anti-inflammatory spices: Add turmeric, ginger, garlic, and fresh herbs like thyme or rosemary for added health benefits and flavor.

Load up on vegetables: Include a variety of colorful vegetables such as carrots, celery, bell peppers, and leafy greens to boost nutritional content.

Choose lean proteins: Opt for lean proteins like chicken breast, turkey, or tofu to add substance without excess fat. Balance flavors: Use a combination of sweet (from vegetables like carrots or sweet potatoes), sour (from tomatoes or citrus), salty (from broth or sea salt), and savory (from herbs and spices) to create a well-rounded flavor profile.

Butternut Squash Soup with Ginger

Servings: 4   Prep Time: 15 minutes   Cook Time: 30 minutes

Ingredients:

- 1 medium butternut squash, peeled, seeded, and diced
- 1 onion, chopped
- 2 cloves garlic, minced
- 1-inch piece fresh ginger, grated
- 4 cups vegetable broth
- 1/2 tsp ground turmeric
- 1/2 tsp ground cinnamon
- Salt and pepper to taste
- 2 tbsp olive oil
- Optional toppings: Greek yogurt, toasted pumpkin seeds, chopped chives

Directions:

1. Heat olive oil in a large pot over medium heat. Add onion and sauté until translucent, about 5 minutes.

2. Add garlic and ginger, and cook for another 1-2 minutes until fragrant.

3. Stir in butternut squash, turmeric, cinnamon, salt, and pepper. Cook for 5 minutes, stirring occasionally.

4. Pour in vegetable broth and bring to a boil. Reduce heat to low, cover, and simmer for 20-25 minutes until squash is tender.

5. Remove from heat and let cool slightly. Blend soup until smooth using an immersion blender or transfer to a blender in batches.

6. Return soup to the pot and reheat if necessary. Adjust seasoning to taste.

7. Serve hot, garnished with Greek yogurt, toasted pumpkin seeds, and chopped chives if desired.

Tips:

- Use pre-cut butternut squash to save time.

- For extra creaminess, add a splash of coconut milk before blending.

- Butternut Squash: Rich in vitamin A, fiber, and antioxidants.

- Ginger and Turmeric: Anti-inflammatory properties.

- Cinnamon: Adds warmth and may help regulate blood sugar levels.

Turmeric Lentil Soup

Servings: 6   Prep Time: 10 minutes

Cook Time: 30 minutes

Ingredients:

- 1 cup dried green lentils, rinsed
- 1 onion, chopped
- 2 carrots, diced
- 2 celery stalks, diced
- 2 cloves garlic, minced
- 1-inch piece fresh ginger, grated
- 1 tsp ground turmeric
- 1 tsp ground cumin
- 6 cups vegetable broth
- Salt and pepper to taste

- 2 tbsp olive oil

- Fresh cilantro or parsley for garnish

Directions:

1. Heat olive oil in a large pot over medium heat. Add onion, carrots, and celery. Sauté until vegetables are tender, about 5-7 minutes.

2. Add garlic, ginger, turmeric, and cumin. Cook for another 1-2 minutes until fragrant.

3. Stir in lentils and vegetable broth. Bring to a boil, then reduce heat to low, cover, and simmer for 20-25 minutes until lentils are tender.

4. Season with salt and pepper to taste.

5. Serve hot, garnished with fresh cilantro or parsley.

Tips:

- Add diced tomatoes for a variation in flavor.

- Blend half of the soup for a creamier texture, if desired.

Nutritional Benefits:

- Lentils: High in protein, fiber, and minerals like iron and folate.

- Turmeric and Cumin: Anti-inflammatory and digestive health benefits.

- Vegetable Broth: Provides vitamins and minerals without added fat.

Chicken and Vegetable Stew

Servings: 4   Prep Time: 15 minutes

Cook Time: 40 minutes

Ingredients:

- 1 lb boneless, skinless chicken breast, cubed
- 1 onion, chopped
- 2 carrots, sliced
- 2 celery stalks, sliced
- 1 bell pepper, diced
- 2 cloves garlic, minced
- 1 tsp dried thyme
- 1 tsp dried rosemary

- 4 cups chicken broth

- 1 cup diced tomatoes (canned or fresh)

- Salt and pepper to taste

- 2 tbsp olive oil

- Fresh parsley for garnish

Directions:

1. Heat olive oil in a large pot over medium heat. Add chicken and cook until browned, about 5-7 minutes. Remove chicken and set aside.

2. In the same pot, add onion, carrots, celery, bell pepper, garlic, thyme, and rosemary. Sauté until vegetables are tender, about 5 minutes.

3. Return chicken to the pot. Add chicken broth and diced tomatoes. Bring to a boil, then reduce heat to low, cover, and simmer for 30 minutes.

4. Season with salt and pepper to taste.

5. Serve hot, garnished with fresh parsley.

Tips:

- Use bone-in chicken for added flavor, removing bones before serving.

- Add spinach or kale for extra greens.

Nutritional Benefits:

- Chicken: Lean protein source.

- Vegetables: Provide vitamins, minerals, and fiber.

- Herbs: Flavorful and contribute antioxidants.

Miso Soup with Seaweed and Tofu

Servings: 4   Prep Time: 10 minutes   Cook Time: 10 minutes

Ingredients:

- 4 cups water
- 4 tbsp white miso paste
- 1 block tofu, cubed
- 1 cup sliced mushrooms (shiitake, button, or any variety)
- 1/2 cup sliced green onions

- 1 sheet nori seaweed, shredded

- 1 tbsp soy sauce or tamari

- 1 tsp sesame oil

- Optional: Sliced chili peppers for heat

Directions:

1. In a pot, bring water to a boil.

2. Reduce heat to low. Add miso paste and stir until dissolved.

3. Add tofu, mushrooms, green onions, and nori seaweed. Simmer for 5-7 minutes until tofu is heated through and mushrooms are tender.

4. Stir in soy sauce or tamari and sesame oil.

5. Taste and adjust seasoning if needed.

6. Serve hot, garnished with sliced chili peppers if desired.

Tips:

- Avoid boiling miso soup once miso paste is added to preserve probiotic benefits.

- Experiment with different types of mushrooms for varied flavors.

Nutritional Benefits:

- Miso Paste: Contains probiotics and offers gut health benefits.

- Tofu: Plant-based protein source.

- Seaweed: Rich in minerals like iodine and supports thyroid health.

Tomato Basil Soup

Servings: 4   Prep Time: 10 minutes   Cook Time: 25 minutes

Ingredients:

- 1 tbsp olive oil
- 1 onion, chopped
- 2 cloves garlic, minced
- 1 tsp dried basil
- 1/2 tsp dried oregano
- 1/4 tsp red pepper flakes (optional)
- 4 cups vegetable broth
- 28 oz canned diced tomatoes
- Salt and pepper to taste

- Fresh basil leaves for garnish

Directions:

1. Heat olive oil in a large pot over medium heat. Add onion and sauté until translucent, about 5-7 minutes.

2. Add garlic, dried basil, oregano, and red pepper flakes (if using). Cook for another 1-2 minutes until fragrant.

3. Pour in vegetable broth and diced tomatoes with their juices. Bring to a boil.

4. Reduce heat to low, cover, and simmer for 15-20 minutes.

5. Use an immersion blender to puree soup until smooth. Alternatively, transfer soup in batches to a blender and blend until smooth. Be cautious with hot liquids.

6. Season with salt and pepper to taste.

7. Serve hot, garnished with fresh basil leaves.

Tips:

- For a creamy texture, stir in a splash of coconut milk or heavy cream before serving.

- Garnish with a drizzle of olive oil and a sprinkle of Parmesan cheese for added flavor.

Nutritional Benefits:

- Tomatoes: Rich in antioxidants like lycopene, which may reduce inflammation.

- Basil: Contains essential oils with potential anti-inflammatory effects.

- Vegetable Broth: Adds depth of flavor without additional calories.

Coconut Curry Soup

Servings: 4   Prep Time: 15 minutes

Cook Time: 25 minutes

Ingredients:

- 1 tbsp coconut oil
- 1 onion, chopped
- 2 cloves garlic, minced
- 1-inch piece fresh ginger, grated
- 1 tbsp curry powder
- 1/2 tsp ground turmeric
- 1/4 tsp cayenne pepper (optional)
- 1 can (14 oz) coconut milk
- 4 cups vegetable broth
- 1 sweet potato, peeled and diced
- 1 red bell pepper, diced
- 1 cup chopped spinach or kale
- Salt and pepper to taste
- Fresh cilantro for garnish

Directions:

1. Heat coconut oil in a large pot over medium heat. Add onion, garlic, and ginger. Sauté until onion is translucent, about 5-7 minutes.

2. Stir in curry powder, turmeric, and cayenne pepper (if using). Cook for another 1-2 minutes until fragrant.

3. Pour in coconut milk and vegetable broth. Bring to a simmer.

4. Add sweet potato and simmer for 10 minutes until tender.

5. Stir in red bell pepper and chopped spinach or kale. Simmer for an additional 5 minutes until vegetables are tender.

6. Season with salt and pepper to taste.

7. Serve hot, garnished with fresh cilantro.

Tips:

- Adjust the level of cayenne pepper for more or less heat.

- Use full-fat coconut milk for a creamier texture and richer flavor.

Nutritional Benefits:

- Coconut Milk: Provides healthy fats and adds creaminess.

- Curry Powder and Turmeric: Anti-inflammatory spices with potential health benefits.

- Sweet Potato and Bell Pepper: Rich in vitamins and antioxidants.

Beef and Barley Stew

Servings: 6   Prep Time: 15 minutes

Cook Time: 1 hour 30 minutes

Ingredients:

- 1 lb beef stew meat, cubed
- 1 onion, chopped
- 2 carrots, sliced
- 2 celery stalks, sliced
- 1 cup pearl barley, rinsed
- 4 cups beef broth
- 1 can (14 oz) diced tomatoes
- 2 tbsp tomato paste
- 2 cloves garlic, minced
- 1 tsp dried thyme

- Salt and pepper to taste
- 2 tbsp olive oil
- Fresh parsley for garnish

Directions:

1. Heat olive oil in a large pot over medium-high heat. Add beef stew meat and cook until browned on all sides, about 5-7 minutes. Remove beef and set aside.

2. In the same pot, add onion, carrots, and celery. Sauté until vegetables are tender, about 5 minutes.

3. Add garlic, thyme, and tomato paste. Cook for another 1-2 minutes until fragrant.

4. Return beef to the pot. Stir in barley, beef broth, and diced tomatoes with their juices. Bring to a boil.

5. Reduce heat to low, cover, and simmer for 1 hour, stirring occasionally, until beef is tender and barley is cooked through.

6. Season with salt and pepper to taste.

7. Serve hot, garnished with fresh parsley.

Tips:

- For a thicker stew, add more tomato paste or simmer uncovered to reduce liquid.

- Make ahead and store in the refrigerator for flavors to meld overnight.

Nutritional Benefits:

- Beef: Provides protein and essential nutrients like iron and zinc.

- Barley: High in fiber and supports digestive health.

- Tomatoes and Vegetables: Rich in vitamins and antioxidants.

Anti-Inflammatory Bone Broth

Servings: Makes about 8 cups   Prep Time: 10 minutes

Cook Time: 12-24 hours

Ingredients:

- 4-5 lbs beef bones (such as marrow bones or knuckles)
- 2 carrots, chopped
- 2 celery stalks, chopped
- 1 onion, quartered
- 4 cloves garlic, smashed
- 2 tbsp apple cider vinegar
- 1 bay leaf
- 1-inch piece fresh ginger (optional)
- Water, enough to cover bones
- Salt and pepper to taste

Directions:

1. Preheat oven to 400°F (200°C). Place beef bones on a baking sheet and roast for 30 minutes until browned.

2. Transfer roasted bones to a large stockpot. Add carrots, celery, onion, garlic, apple cider vinegar, bay leaf, and ginger (if using).

3. Pour enough water to cover bones and vegetables.

4. Bring to a boil over high heat, then reduce heat to low. Simmer, uncovered, for 12-24 hours, skimming any foam that rises to the top.

5. Strain bone broth through a fine-mesh sieve or cheesecloth into a clean container. Discard solids.

6. Season with salt and pepper to taste.

7. Let bone broth cool before refrigerating or freezing in portions.

Tips:

- Use organic ingredients for maximum nutritional benefits.

- Drink bone broth on its own or use it as a base for soups and stews.

Nutritional Benefits:

- Bone Broth: Rich in collagen, amino acids, and minerals that support gut health and joint function.

- Vegetables: Provide vitamins and antioxidants.

- Apple Cider Vinegar: Helps extract nutrients from bones.

Spicy Black Bean Soup

Servings: 6   Prep Time: 10 minutes

Cook Time: 30 minutes

Ingredients:

- 2 cans (15 oz each) black beans, rinsed and drained
- 1 onion, chopped
- 2 cloves garlic, minced
- 1 red bell pepper, diced
- 1 jalapeño pepper, seeded and minced
- 1 tsp ground cumin
- 1 tsp smoked paprika
- 4 cups vegetable broth
- Juice of 1 lime
- Salt and pepper to taste
- 2 tbsp olive oil

- Fresh cilantro for garnish

- Optional toppings: Greek yogurt, avocado slices, tortilla strips

Directions:

1. Heat olive oil in a large pot over medium heat. Add onion, garlic, red bell pepper, and jalapeño pepper. Sauté until vegetables are tender, about 5-7 minutes.

2. Stir in ground cumin and smoked paprika. Cook for another 1-2 minutes until fragrant.

3. Add black beans and vegetable broth. Bring to a boil, then reduce heat to low, cover, and simmer for 20 minutes.

4. Use an immersion blender to partially blend soup until desired consistency. Alternatively, transfer half of the soup to a blender and blend until smooth, then return to the pot.

5. Stir in lime juice. Season with salt and pepper to taste.

6. Serve hot, garnished with fresh cilantro and your choice of toppings.

Tips:

- For a creamier soup, blend all of the soup until smooth.

- Adjust spiciness by adding more or less jalapeño pepper.

Nutritional Benefits:

- Black Beans: High in protein and fiber, supports digestive health.

- Bell Pepper and Jalapeño: Rich in vitamins and antioxidants.

- Lime Juice: Adds a refreshing citrus flavor and provides vitamin C.

Carrot Ginger Soup

Servings: 4   Prep Time: 10 minutes

Cook Time: 25 minutes

Ingredients:

- 1 tbsp coconut oil or olive oil
- 1 onion, chopped
- 1 lb carrots, peeled and chopped
- 2 cloves garlic, minced
- 1-inch piece fresh ginger, grated
- 4 cups vegetable broth
- 1 can (14 oz) coconut milk
- Salt and pepper to taste

- Fresh cilantro or parsley for garnish

Directions:

1. Heat coconut oil or olive oil in a large pot over medium heat. Add onion and sauté until translucent, about 5-7 minutes.

2. Add carrots, garlic, and ginger. Cook for another 1-2 minutes until fragrant.

3. Pour in vegetable broth and bring to a boil. Reduce heat to low, cover, and simmer for 15-20 minutes until carrots are tender.

4. Use an immersion blender to puree soup until smooth. Alternatively, transfer soup in batches to a blender and blend until smooth. Be cautious with hot liquids.

5. Stir in coconut milk. Season with salt and pepper to taste.

6. Serve hot, garnished with fresh cilantro or parsley.

Tips:

- Adjust the consistency by adding more vegetable broth or coconut milk.

- For extra creaminess, stir in a tablespoon of almond butter before blending.

Nutritional Benefits:

- Carrots: High in beta-carotene and fiber.

- Ginger: Anti-inflammatory properties and aids digestion.

- Coconut Milk: Adds creaminess and healthy fats.

Chapter 7: Anti-Inflammatory Desserts Without the Guilt

"You don't have to give up dessert to eat healthy." - Unknown

In this chapter, we explore the delightful world of desserts that not only satisfy your sweet tooth but also support your anti-inflammatory diet goals. You'll discover how to use wholesome ingredients to create treats that are both delicious and beneficial for your health.

Creating Delicious and Healthy Desserts:

- Discuss the myth that desserts must be unhealthy and explore the possibility of using natural, anti-inflammatory ingredients to create guilt-free treats.

- Highlight the importance of moderation and balance in enjoying desserts while following an anti-inflammatory lifestyle.

Using Anti-Inflammatory Ingredients in Sweets:

- Introduction to key anti-inflammatory ingredients commonly used in desserts, such as berries, nuts, dark chocolate, and spices like cinnamon and ginger.

- Explain the health benefits of these ingredients and how they can reduce inflammation in the body.

Berry Chia Seed Pudding

Servings: 4   Prep Time: 10 minutes

(+2 hours chilling time)

Ingredients:

- 1 cup mixed berries (such as strawberries, blueberries, raspberries)
- 1/4 cup chia seeds
- 1 cup unsweetened almond milk
- 1 tbsp maple syrup (optional, adjust to taste)
- 1/2 tsp vanilla extract

Directions:

1. In a blender, combine mixed berries, almond milk, maple syrup (if using), and vanilla extract. Blend until smooth.

2. Pour the berry mixture into a bowl. Stir in chia seeds until well combined.

3. Cover and refrigerate for at least 2 hours or overnight, until the chia seeds have absorbed the liquid and the mixture has thickened.

4. Stir well before serving. Divide into bowls and top with additional berries if desired.

Tips:

- Use your favorite berries for variety and additional antioxidants.

- Adjust sweetness with more or less maple syrup, or substitute with honey or agave syrup.

Nutritional Benefits:

- Berries: Packed with antioxidants and vitamins.

- Chia Seeds: High in omega-3 fatty acids and fiber.

- Almond Milk: Provides calcium and vitamin E without dairy.

Dark Chocolate Avocado Mousse

Servings: 4   Prep Time: 10 minutes (+1 hour chilling time)

Ingredients:

- 2 ripe avocados, peeled and pitted
- 1/4 cup unsweetened cocoa powder
- 1/4 cup maple syrup or honey
- 1 tsp vanilla extract
- Pinch of salt
- Fresh berries for garnish

Directions:

1. In a food processor or blender, combine avocados, cocoa powder, maple syrup or honey, vanilla extract, and salt. Blend until smooth and creamy.

2. Taste and adjust sweetness if needed.

3. Transfer the mousse into serving bowls or glasses.

4. Cover and refrigerate for at least 1 hour to chill and firm up.

5. Before serving, garnish with fresh berries.

Tips:

- Use ripe avocados for a creamy texture and natural sweetness.

- Add a sprinkle of sea salt or a dash of cinnamon for extra flavor.

Nutritional Benefits:

- Avocados: Healthy fats and fiber.

- Dark Chocolate: Contains antioxidants and may lower inflammation markers.

Turmeric Ginger Lemon Cookies

Servings: 12 cookies   Prep Time: 15 minutes

Cook Time: 12-15 minutes

Ingredients:

- 1 cup almond flour
- 1/4 cup coconut flour
- 1 tsp ground turmeric
- 1 tsp ground ginger
- 1/2 tsp baking powder

- Pinch of salt

- 1/4 cup coconut oil, melted

- 1/4 cup maple syrup or honey

- Zest of 1 lemon

- 1 tbsp fresh lemon juice

Directions:

1. Preheat oven to 350°F (175°C). Line a baking sheet with parchment paper.

2. In a mixing bowl, whisk together almond flour, coconut flour, turmeric, ginger, baking powder, and salt.

3. In a separate bowl, whisk together melted coconut oil, maple syrup or honey, lemon zest, and lemon juice.

4. Add wet ingredients to dry ingredients and stir until well combined.

5. Roll dough into tablespoon-sized balls and place them on the prepared baking sheet. Flatten each ball slightly with the palm of your hand.

6. Bake for 12-15 minutes, until edges are golden brown.

7. Remove from oven and let cool on the baking sheet for 5 minutes, then transfer to a wire rack to cool completely.

Tips:

- Adjust spices to your preference for more or less ginger and turmeric flavor.

- Store cookies in an airtight container for up to 5 days.

Nutritional Benefits:

- Almond Flour and Coconut Flour: Gluten-free alternatives rich in healthy fats and fiber.

- Turmeric and Ginger: Anti-inflammatory spices with potential health benefits.

- Lemon: Provides vitamin C and adds brightness to the cookies.

Coconut Yogurt Parfait with Fresh Fruit

Servings: 2   Prep Time: 10 minutes

Ingredients:

- 1 cup unsweetened coconut yogurt
- 1 cup mixed fresh berries (such as strawberries, blueberries, raspberries)
- 1/4 cup granola (choose a variety without added sugars)
- 2 tbsp shredded coconut (optional)

Directions:

1. In two serving glasses or bowls, layer coconut yogurt, mixed berries, and granola.

2. Repeat layers until glasses are filled.

3. Top with shredded coconut if using.

4. Serve immediately.

Tips:

- Use dairy-free coconut yogurt for a plant-based option.

- Experiment with different fruits and granola flavors for variety.

Nutritional Benefits:

- Coconut Yogurt: Provides probiotics and healthy fats.

- Berries: Antioxidant-rich and low in calories.

- Granola: Adds crunch and fiber, choose a variety with minimal added sugars.

Spiced Poached Pears

Servings: 4   Prep Time: 10 minutes

Cook Time: 20 minutes

Ingredients:

- 4 ripe pears, peeled and halved
- 2 cups water
- 1/2 cup orange juice
- 1/4 cup honey or maple syrup
- 1 cinnamon stick
- 4 whole cloves
- 1-inch piece fresh ginger, sliced

Directions:

1. In a large saucepan, combine water, orange juice, honey or maple syrup, cinnamon stick, cloves, and ginger. Bring to a boil.

2. Reduce heat to low and add pear halves, cut side down. Simmer gently for 15-20 minutes, until pears are tender but not mushy, turning occasionally.

3. Remove pears with a slotted spoon and transfer to serving plates or bowls.

4. Increase heat to medium-high and boil the poaching liquid until reduced by half, about 10 minutes.

5. Remove from heat and discard cinnamon stick, cloves, and ginger slices.

6. Spoon the reduced poaching liquid over the pears.

7. Serve warm or chilled.

Tips:

- Choose firm pears that will hold their shape during poaching.

- Serve with a dollop of Greek yogurt or a sprinkle of chopped nuts for added texture.

- Pears: High in fiber and vitamin C.

- Spices: Cinnamon, cloves, and ginger offer anti-inflammatory properties.

- Orange Juice: Adds sweetness and vitamin C.

Turmeric Mango Sorbet

Servings: 4   Prep Time: 10 minutes (+ freezing time)

Ingredients:

- 2 cups frozen mango chunks
- 1/2 cup coconut milk
- 1 tbsp fresh lime juice
- 1 tsp ground turmeric
- 2 tbsp honey or maple syrup (optional, adjust to taste)
- Fresh mint leaves for garn

Directions:

1. In a blender or food processor, combine frozen mango chunks, coconut milk, lime juice, turmeric, and honey or maple syrup (if using).

2. Blend until smooth and creamy, scraping down the sides as needed.

3. Taste and adjust sweetness or turmeric amount if desired.

4. Transfer the sorbet mixture into a freezer-safe container. Cover and freeze for at least 4 hours or until firm.

5. Before serving, let the sorbet sit at room temperature for a few minutes to soften slightly.

6. Scoop into bowls or cones, garnish with fresh mint leaves, and enjoy immediately.

Tips:

- Use ripe and sweet mangoes for the best flavor.

- Add a pinch of black pepper when blending to enhance the absorption of turmeric's benefits.

Nutritional Benefits:

- Mango: High in vitamins A and C, antioxidants, and fiber.

- Coconut Milk: Provides healthy fats and a creamy texture.

- Turmeric: Anti-inflammatory properties and adds vibrant color.

Chia Seed Pudding with Berries

Servings: 2   Prep Time: 5 minutes
(+2 hours chilling time)

Ingredients:

- 1/4 cup chia seeds
- 1 cup unsweetened almond milk (or any milk of choice)
- 1/2 tsp vanilla extract
- 1 tbsp honey or maple syrup (optional, adjust to taste)
- 1/2 cup mixed berries (such as strawberries, blueberries, raspberries)
- Fresh mint leaves for garnish

Directions:

1. In a bowl, whisk together chia seeds, almond milk, vanilla extract, and honey or maple syrup (if using). Stir well to combine.

2. Cover the bowl and refrigerate for at least 2 hours or overnight, until the chia seeds have absorbed the liquid and the mixture has thickened.

3. Stir the chia pudding before serving to break up any clumps.

4. Divide the pudding into serving bowls or jars.

5. Top with mixed berries and garnish with fresh mint leaves.

6. Serve chilled.

Tips:

- Experiment with different toppings such as nuts, seeds, or coconut flakes.

- Adjust sweetness by adding more or less honey or maple syrup.

Nutritional Benefits:

- Chia Seeds: High in omega-3 fatty acids, fiber, and protein.

- Berries: Rich in antioxidants, vitamins, and minerals.

- Almond Milk: Provides calcium and vitamin E without dairy.

Dark Chocolate Avocado Mousse

Servings: 4   Prep Time: 10 minutes

(+1 hour chilling time)

Ingredients:

- 2 ripe avocados, peeled and pitted
- 1/4 cup unsweetened cocoa powder
- 1/4 cup maple syrup or honey
- 1 tsp vanilla extract
- Pinch of salt
- Fresh berries for garnish

Directions:

1. In a food processor or blender, combine avocados, cocoa powder, maple syrup or honey, vanilla extract, and salt. Blend until smooth and creamy.

2. Taste and adjust sweetness if needed.

3. Transfer the mousse into serving bowls or glasses.

4. Cover and refrigerate for at least 1 hour to chill and firm up.

5. Before serving, garnish with fresh berries.

Tips:

- Use ripe avocados for a creamy texture and natural sweetness.

- Add a sprinkle of sea salt or a dash of cinnamon for extra flavor.

Nutritional Benefits:

- Avocados: Healthy fats and fiber.

- Dark Chocolate: Contains antioxidants and may lower inflammation markers.

- Maple Syrup or Honey: Natural sweeteners with potential health benefits compared to refined sugar.

Coconut Macaroons

Servings: 12-15 macaroons   Prep Time: 10 minutes

Cook Time: 15 minutes

Ingredients:

- 2 cups shredded unsweetened coconut

- 1/3 cup coconut flour

- 1/2 cup coconut oil, melted

- 1/2 cup honey or maple syrup

- 1 tsp vanilla extract

- Pinch of salt

- Optional: Dark chocolate for drizzling

- Directions:

1. Preheat oven to 325°F (160°C). Line a baking sheet with parchment paper.

2. In a large bowl, combine shredded coconut, coconut flour, melted coconut oil, honey or maple syrup, vanilla extract, and salt. Mix until well combined.

3. Scoop tablespoon-sized portions of the mixture and roll into balls. Place them on the prepared baking sheet.

4. Bake for 12-15 minutes, until edges are golden brown.

5. Remove from the oven and let cool completely on the baking sheet.

6. Optional: Melt dark chocolate and drizzle over cooled macaroons for added flavor.

7. Allow chocolate to set before serving or storing.

Tips:

- Adjust sweetness by adding more or less honey or maple syrup.

- Store macaroons in an airtight container at room temperature for up to one week.

Nutritional Benefits:

- Coconut: Provides healthy fats and adds flavor and texture.

- Coconut Oil: Contains medium-chain triglycerides (MCTs) with potential health benefits.

- Honey or Maple Syrup: Natural sweeteners with antioxidants and minerals.

Almond Flour Brownies

Servings: 12 brownies   Prep Time: 10 minutes   Cook Time: 25-30 minutes

Ingredients:

- 1 cup almond flour
- 1/2 cup cocoa powder
- 1/2 tsp baking soda
- 1/4 tsp salt
- 1/2 cup coconut oil, melted
- 1/2 cup honey or maple syrup
- 2 eggs
- 1 tsp vanilla extract
- 1/2 cup dark chocolate chips (optional)

Directions:

1. Preheat oven to 350°F (175°C). Grease or line an 8x8-inch baking pan with parchment paper.

2. In a large bowl, whisk together almond flour, cocoa powder, baking soda, and salt.

3. In a separate bowl, whisk together melted coconut oil, honey or maple syrup, eggs, and vanilla extract until smooth.

4. Pour wet ingredients into dry ingredients and stir until well combined.

5. Fold in dark chocolate chips if using.

6. Pour batter into the prepared baking pan and spread evenly.

7. Bake for 25-30 minutes, until edges are set and a toothpick inserted into the center comes out with moist crumbs.

8. Remove from oven and let cool completely in the pan on a wire rack before slicing into squares.

Tips:

- Use high-quality cocoa powder for rich chocolate flavor.

- For fudgier brownies, slightly underbake and let cool completely before cutting.

Nutritional Benefits:

- Almond Flour: Gluten-free alternative with healthy fats and protein.

- Dark Chocolate: Contains antioxidants and may support heart health.

- Coconut Oil: Adds moisture and beneficial fats.

Apple Cinnamon Baked Apples

Servings: 4   Prep Time: 15 minutes   Cook Time: 25-30 minutes

Ingredients:

- 4 large apples (such as Honeycrisp or Fuji)
- 1/2 cup chopped nuts (such as walnuts or almonds)
- 1/4 cup dried cranberries or raisins
- 2 tbsp honey or maple syrup
- 1 tsp ground cinnamon
- 1/4 tsp ground nutmeg
- 1/4 tsp vanilla extract
- 1/2 cup water or apple juice

Directions:

1. Preheat oven to 375°F (190°C). Grease a baking dish large enough to hold the apples.

2. Core the apples using an apple corer or a small knife, leaving the bottom intact to create a cavity.

3. In a small bowl, combine chopped nuts, dried cranberries or raisins, honey or maple syrup, cinnamon, nutmeg, and vanilla extract. Mix well.

4. Stuff each apple with the nut mixture, pressing gently to fill the cavity.

5. Place stuffed apples in the prepared baking dish. Pour water or apple juice into the bottom of the dish.

6. Cover the baking dish with foil and bake for 20 minutes.

7. Remove foil and bake for an additional 5-10 minutes, until apples are tender and filling is bubbly.

8. Remove from oven and let cool slightly before serving.

Tips:

- Serve baked apples warm with a dollop of Greek yogurt or a scoop of vanilla ice cream.

- Experiment with different nuts and dried fruits for variety.

Nutritional Benefits:

- Apples: High in fiber and vitamin C.

- Nuts: Provide healthy fats, protein, and essential nutrients.

- Cinnamon: Adds warmth and may have anti-inflammatory properties.

Matcha Green Tea Ice Cream

Servings: 4   Prep Time: 10 minutes (+2 hours chilling time)

Ingredients:

- 1 can (14 oz) full-fat coconut milk, chilled
- 2-3 tbsp matcha green tea powder
- 1/4 cup honey or maple syrup
- 1 tsp vanilla extract
- Optional: Dark chocolate shavings for garnish

Directions:

1. Chill the can of coconut milk in the refrigerator overnight.

2. Open the can of coconut milk and scoop out the thick cream that has risen to the top (save the coconut water for another use).

3. In a bowl, whisk together coconut cream, matcha green tea powder, honey or maple syrup, and vanilla extract until smooth and well combined.

4. Taste and adjust sweetness or matcha powder amount if desired.

5. Pour the mixture into a freezer-safe container.

6. Cover and freeze for about 2 hours, stirring every 30 minutes to break up any ice crystals.

7. Once the ice cream is firm but scoopable, serve immediately.

8. Garnish with dark chocolate shavings if desired.

Tips:

- Use high-quality matcha powder for vibrant color and flavor.

- For a creamier texture, use an ice cream maker if available.

- Matcha Green Tea: Contains antioxidants and may promote relaxation and focus.

- Coconut Milk: Provides healthy fats and a creamy base without dairy.

- Honey or Maple Syrup: Natural sweeteners with potential health benefits compared to refined sugar.

Pumpkin Spice Energy Balls

Servings: 12-15 energy balls   Prep Time: 15 minutes (+30 minutes chilling time)

Ingredients:

- 1 cup rolled oats
- 1/2 cup pumpkin puree
- 1/4 cup almond butter
- 1/4 cup honey or maple syrup
- 1 tsp vanilla extract
- 1 tsp ground cinnamon
- 1/2 tsp ground nutmeg
- 1/4 tsp ground ginger
- Pinch of salt
- 1/2 cup shredded coconut (optional, for rolling)

Directions:

1. In a food processor, combine rolled oats, pumpkin puree, almond butter, honey or maple syrup, vanilla extract, cinnamon, nutmeg, ginger, and salt. Pulse until mixture is well combined and forms a sticky dough.

2. Scoop tablespoon-sized portions of the mixture and roll into balls.

3. If desired, roll each ball in shredded coconut to coat.

4. Place energy balls on a baking sheet lined with parchment paper.

5. Chill in the refrigerator for at least 30 minutes to firm up.

6. Store energy balls in an airtight container in the refrigerator for up to one week.

Tips:

- Adjust sweetness or spice levels according to your preference.

- Add chopped nuts or dried fruits for extra texture and flavor.

Nutritional Benefits:

- Pumpkin Puree: Rich in vitamins A and C, fiber, and antioxidants.

- Almond Butter: Provides protein, healthy fats, and vitamin E.

- Oats: Source of fiber and complex carbohydrates for sustained energy.

Lemon Poppy Seed Muffins

Servings: 12 muffins

Prep Time: 15 minutes

Cook Time: 20-25 minutes

Ingredients:

- 2 cups almond flour
- 1/4 cup coconut flour
- 1/2 tsp baking soda
- 1/4 tsp salt
- Zest of 2 lemons
- Juice of 1 lemon
- 1/3 cup honey or maple syrup
- 1/4 cup coconut oil, melted
- 3 eggs
- 1 tsp vanilla extract
- 2 tbsp poppy seeds

Directions:

1. Preheat oven to 350°F (175°C). Line a muffin tin with paper liners or grease with coconut oil.

2. In a large bowl, whisk together almond flour, coconut flour, baking soda, salt, and lemon zest.

3. In a separate bowl, whisk together lemon juice, honey or maple syrup, melted coconut oil, eggs, and vanilla extract.

4. Pour wet ingredients into dry ingredients and stir until just combined.

5. Gently fold in poppy seeds.

6. Spoon batter evenly into muffin cups, filling each about 3/4 full.

7. Bake for 20-25 minutes, until muffins are golden brown and a toothpick inserted into the center comes out clean.

8. Remove from oven and let cool in the pan for 5 minutes, then transfer to a wire rack to cool completely.

Tips:

- Add a lemon glaze or drizzle for extra sweetness.

- Store muffins in an airtight container at room temperature for up to 3 days, or refrigerate for longer freshness.

- Almond Flour and Coconut Flour: Gluten-free alternatives with healthy fats and protein.

- Lemon: Provides vitamin C and adds bright flavor.

- Poppy Seeds: Source of fiber, essential minerals, and antioxidants.

Banana Oat Cookies

Servings: 12-15 cookies   Prep Time: 10 minutes

Cook Time: 15-18 minutes

Ingredients:

- 2 ripe bananas, mashed
- 1 1/2 cups rolled oats
- 1/4 cup almond flour
- 1/4 cup coconut oil, melted
- 1/4 cup honey or maple syrup
- 1 tsp vanilla extract
- 1/2 tsp ground cinnamon
- Pinch of salt

- 1/2 cup dark chocolate chips or chopped nuts (optional)

1. Preheat oven to 350°F (175°C). Line a baking sheet with parchment paper.

2. In a large bowl, combine mashed bananas, rolled oats, almond flour, melted coconut oil, honey or maple syrup, vanilla extract, cinnamon, and salt. Mix until well combined.

3. If using, fold in dark chocolate chips or chopped nuts.

4. Drop spoonfuls of cookie dough onto the prepared baking sheet, spacing them slightly apart.

5. Flatten each cookie with the back of a spoon or your fingers.

6. Bake for 15-18 minutes, until edges are golden brown.

7. Remove from oven and let cool on the baking sheet for 5 minutes, then transfer to a wire rack to cool completely.

Tips:

- Customize cookies with your favorite add-ins like dried fruits or seeds.

- Store cookies in an airtight container at room temperature for up to 5 days.

Nutritional Benefits:

- Bananas: Provide natural sweetness and potassium.

- Oats and Almond Flour: Source of fiber, protein, and healthy fats.

- Coconut Oil: Adds moisture and beneficial fats.

Chapter 8: Anti-Inflammatory Meals for Special Occasions

"Special occasions call for special meals that nourish the body and soul." - Unknown

Special occasions often bring indulgent feasts, but they don't have to derail your health goals. With a bit of planning, you can create meals that are both festive and anti-inflammatory. Whether it's a holiday gathering, a birthday celebration, or a family reunion, these recipes will ensure that your meals are as nourishing as they are delicious. Balancing indulgence and nutrition is key, and with the right ingredients and preparation techniques, you can enjoy the festivities without compromising on health. Dive into these recipes designed for memorable occasions and discover how to make every celebration both joyful and health-conscious..

. Roasted Turkey with Herb Rub

Servings: 8-10   Prep Time: 30 minutes   Cook Time: 3-4 hours

Ingredients:

- 1 whole turkey (10-12 pounds)
- 1/2 cup olive oil or melted ghee
- 1/4 cup fresh rosemary, chopped
- 1/4 cup fresh thyme, chopped
- 1/4 cup fresh sage, chopped
- 4 cloves garlic, minced
- 1 lemon, halved
- Salt and pepper to taste

Directions:

1. Preheat oven to 325°F (165°C).

2. In a bowl, mix olive oil or melted ghee, rosemary, thyme, sage, garlic, salt, and pepper.

3. Pat the turkey dry with paper towels. Rub the herb mixture all over the turkey, including under the skin.

4. Place the lemon halves inside the turkey cavity.

5. Place the turkey on a roasting rack in a large roasting pan.

6. Roast the turkey for 3-4 hours, or until a meat thermometer reads 165°F (75°C) when inserted into the thickest part of the thigh.

7. Let the turkey rest for 20 minutes before carving.

Tips:

- Baste the turkey every hour with the pan juices for a moist and flavorful bird.

- Save the turkey bones to make a nourishing bone broth.

Nutritional Benefits:

- Turkey: A lean source of protein and rich in B vitamins.

- Herbs: Packed with antioxidants and anti-inflammatory properties.

Stuffed Acorn Squash

Servings: 4   Prep Time: 20 minutes   Cook Time: 1 hour

Ingredients:

- 2 acorn squash, halved and seeded
- 1 cup quinoa, cooked
- 1/2 cup dried cranberries
- 1/2 cup chopped pecans
- 1/4 cup fresh parsley, chopped
- 1/2 tsp ground cinnamon
- 2 tbsp olive oil
- Salt and pepper to taste

Directions:

1. Preheat oven to 375°F (190°C).

2. Brush the squash halves with olive oil, and season with salt and pepper.

3. Place the squash halves cut-side down on a baking sheet and roast for 30 minutes.

4. In a bowl, mix the cooked quinoa, cranberries, pecans, parsley, cinnamon, and a tablespoon of olive oil.

5. Remove the squash from the oven and fill each half with the quinoa mixture.

6. Return to the oven and bake for an additional 20 minutes.

Tips:

- Substitute cranberries with raisins or dried cherries for a different flavor.

- Add a sprinkle of feta cheese before serving for added richness.

Nutritional Benefits:

- Acorn Squash: High in vitamins A and C, and fiber.

- Quinoa: A complete protein and rich in minerals.

Holiday Spiced Cranberry Sauce

Servings: 8   Prep Time: 10 minutes   Cook Time: 20 minutes

Ingredients:

- 12 oz fresh cranberries
- 1/2 cup honey or maple syrup
- 1/2 cup orange juice
- 1 tsp ground cinnamon
- 1/4 tsp ground nutmeg
- 1/4 tsp ground cloves

Directions:

1. In a saucepan, combine cranberries, honey or maple syrup, orange juice, cinnamon, nutmeg, and cloves.

2. Bring to a boil over medium heat, then reduce to a simmer.

3. Cook, stirring occasionally, until the cranberries burst and the sauce thickens, about 15-20 minutes.

4. Let cool before serving.

Tips:

- Make this sauce a day ahead to allow flavors to meld.

- Add a splash of brandy or port wine for an adult twist.

Nutritional Benefits:

- Cranberries: Rich in antioxidants and support urinary tract health.

- Honey: Contains antioxidants and has anti-inflammatory properties.

Garlic Rosemary Mashed Cauliflower

Servings: 4   Prep Time: 10 minutes   Cook Time: 20 minutes

Ingredients:

- 1 large head of cauliflower, cut into florets
- 3 cloves garlic, minced
- 2 tbsp olive oil
- 1/4 cup unsweetened almond milk
- 2 tbsp fresh rosemary, chopped
- Salt and pepper to taste

Directions:

1. Steam the cauliflower florets until tender, about 10-12 minutes.

2. In a skillet, sauté garlic in olive oil until fragrant.

3. In a food processor, combine steamed cauliflower, sautéed garlic, almond milk, rosemary, salt, and pepper. Blend until smooth and creamy.

4. Adjust seasoning to taste.

- For extra creaminess, add a dollop of Greek yogurt or sour cream.

- Top with chopped chives or a drizzle of truffle oil for added flavor.

Nutritional Benefits:

- Cauliflower: High in fiber, vitamins C and K, and has anti-inflammatory effects.

- Garlic: Contains compounds with potent medicinal properties.

Maple Glazed Carrots

Servings: 4   Prep Time: 10 minutes

Cook Time: 25 minutes

Ingredients:

- 1 pound carrots, peeled and sliced
- 2 tbsp olive oil
- 2 tbsp pure maple syrup
- 1 tsp ground cinnamon
- Salt and pepper to taste

Directions:

1. Preheat oven to 400°F (200°C).

2. In a bowl, toss the carrots with olive oil, maple syrup, cinnamon, salt, and pepper.

3. Spread the carrots on a baking sheet in a single layer.

4. Roast for 25 minutes, or until tender and caramelized, stirring halfway through.

Tips:

- Add a sprinkle of chopped fresh parsley before serving for color and freshness.

- Use rainbow carrots for a visually appealing dish.

Nutritional Benefits:

- Carrots: High in beta-carotene, fiber, and antioxidants.

- Maple Syrup: Natural sweetener with a lower glycemic index than refined sugar.

Quinoa Stuffing with Apples and Pecans

Servings: 6

Prep Time: 15 minutes

Cook Time: 20 minutes

Ingredients:

- 1 cup quinoa, rinsed and cooked
- 1 apple, diced
- 1/2 cup pecans, chopped
- 1/4 cup dried cranberries
- 1 small onion, finely chopped
- 2 celery stalks, chopped
- 2 tbsp olive oil
- 1 tsp dried sage
- 1/2 tsp dried thyme
- Salt and pepper to taste

Directions:

1. In a skillet, heat olive oil over medium heat. Sauté onion and celery until softened.

2. Add the apple and cook for 3-4 minutes.

3. Stir in cooked quinoa, pecans, cranberries, sage, thyme, salt, and pepper.

4. Cook until heated through, about 5 minutes.

Tips:

- Use vegetable broth instead of water for cooking quinoa for added flavor.

- Add cooked sausage for a heartier stuffing.

Nutritional Benefits:

- Quinoa: Complete protein and rich in minerals.

- Apples: Provide fiber, vitamins, and antioxidants.

Herbed Salmon with Citrus Glaze

Servings: 4   Prep Time: 10 minutes   Cook Time: 15 minutes

Ingredients:

- 4 salmon fillets
- 2 tbsp olive oil
- 1 lemon, thinly sliced
- 1 orange, thinly sliced
- 2 tbsp fresh dill, chopped
- 2 tbsp fresh parsley, chopped
- Salt and pepper to taste

Directions:

1. Preheat oven to 375°F (190°C).

2. Place salmon fillets on a baking sheet lined with parchment paper.

3. Drizzle olive oil over the fillets and season with salt and pepper.

4. Arrange lemon and orange slices on top of the salmon.

5. Sprinkle with dill and parsley.

6. Bake for 12-15 minutes, until salmon is cooked through and flakes easily with a fork.

Tips:

- Serve with a side of roasted vegetables or a fresh salad.

- Use leftover salmon in salads or sandwiches the next day.

Nutritional Benefits:

- Salmon: Rich in omega-3 fatty acids, protein, and vitamin D.

- Citrus Fruits: Provide vitamin C and antioxidants.

Pumpkin Soup with Sage

Servings: 4   Prep Time: 10 minutes   Cook Time: 20 minutes

Ingredients:

- 4 cups pumpkin puree
- 1 small onion, chopped
- 2 cloves garlic, minced
- 2 cups vegetable broth
- 1 cup coconut milk
- 1 tbsp olive oil
- 1 tsp ground cinnamon
- 1/2 tsp ground nutmeg
- 1/4 tsp ground ginger
- Salt and pepper to taste
- 1 tbsp fresh sage, chopped

Directions:

1. In a large pot, heat olive oil over medium heat. Sauté onion and garlic until translucent.

2. Add pumpkin puree, vegetable broth, coconut milk, cinnamon, nutmeg, ginger, salt, and pepper. Stir to combine.

3. Bring to a boil, then reduce heat and simmer for 15 minutes.

4. Use an immersion blender to puree the soup until smooth.

5. Stir in chopped sage and adjust seasoning as needed.

Tips:

- Serve with a dollop of Greek yogurt or a sprinkle of pumpkin seeds.

- Use fresh pumpkin for a more robust flavor.

Nutritional Benefits:

- Pumpkin: High in vitamins A and C, and antioxidants.

- Sage: Contains anti-inflammatory and antioxidant properties.

Festive Beet and Goat Cheese Salad

Servings: 4   Prep Time: 15 minutes   Cook Time: 45 minutes

Ingredients:

- 4 medium beets, roasted and sliced
- 4 oz goat cheese, crumbled
- 1/4 cup walnuts, toasted
- 4 cups mixed greens
- 2 tbsp olive oil
- 1 tbsp balsamic vinegar
- Salt and pepper to taste

Directions:

1. Preheat oven to 400°F (200°C). Wrap beets in foil and roast for 45 minutes, or until tender. Let cool, then peel and slice.

2. In a large bowl, combine mixed greens, roasted beets, goat cheese, and walnuts.

3. In a small bowl, whisk together olive oil, balsamic vinegar, salt, and pepper.

4. Drizzle the dressing over the salad and toss to combine.

Tips:

- Add a sprinkle of pomegranate seeds for extra festive color and flavor.

- Use arugula for a peppery twist.

Nutritional Benefits:

- Beets: High in fiber, vitamins, and antioxidants.

- Goat Cheese: Contains protein and calcium.

Dark Chocolate Bark with Nuts and Berries

Servings: 8   Prep Time: 10 minutes   Cook Time: 10 minutes (plus cooling time)

Ingredients:

- 8 oz dark chocolate (70% cocoa or higher)
- 1/4 cup almonds, chopped
- 1/4 cup pistachios, chopped
- 1/4 cup dried cranberries
- 1/4 cup dried blueberries
- 1/4 tsp sea salt

Directions:

1. Melt the dark chocolate in a double boiler or microwave, stirring until smooth.

2. Line a baking sheet with parchment paper.

3. Pour the melted chocolate onto the parchment paper and spread into an even layer.

4. Sprinkle almonds, pistachios, cranberries, blueberries, and sea salt over the chocolate.

5. Let the chocolate cool and harden at room temperature, or refrigerate for faster results.

6. Once set, break into pieces and serve.

Tips:

- Store the chocolate bark in an airtight container for up to a week.

- Experiment with different nuts and dried fruits for variety.

Nutritional Benefits:

- Dark Chocolate: Rich in antioxidants and can improve heart health.

- Nuts and Berries: Provide healthy fats, fiber, vitamins, and minerals.